How Many Nurses Do I Need?
A Guide to Resource Management Issues

Edited by Lynn M. Dunne

A collection of articles first published in *Professional Nurse* and here revised and updated, with additional articles specially commissioned for inclusion

Wolfe Publishing Ltd

Published by
Wolfe Publishing Ltd
Brook House
2–16 Torrington Place
London WC1E 7LT

Printed by BPCC Hazell Books, Aylesbury, England.

For full details of all Wolfe Nursing titles please write to Wolfe
Publishing Ltd, Brook House, 2–16 Torrington Place, London
WC1E 7LT, England.

How Many Nurses Do I Need?
A Guide to Resource Management Issues

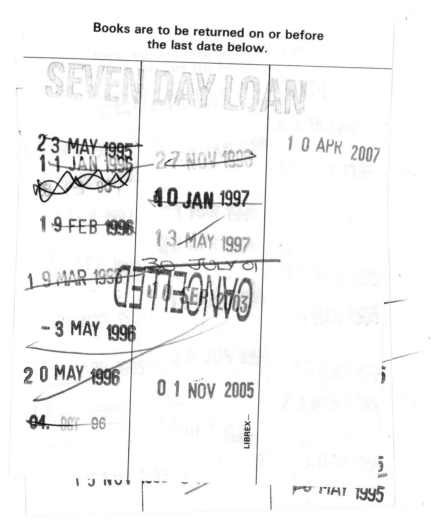

The Professional Developments Series

These eight books provide you with a wealth of insight into all aspects of nursing practice. The series is essential reading for qualified, practising nurses who need to keep up-to-date with new developments, evaluate their clinical practice, and develop and extend their clinical management and teaching skills. Through reading these books, students of nursing will gain an insight into what the essence of nursing is and the wide range of skills which are daily employed in improving patient care. Up-to-date, referenced and appropriately illustrated, The Professional Developments Series brings together the work of well over two hundred nurses.

Other titles in The Professional Developments Series:

Garrett   **Healthy Ageing: Some Nursing Perspectives**   1 870065 22 0
This book puts healthy ageing into the context of a growing, healthy elderly population and looks at care aspects of daily living, health problems in old age, and working with older people.

Glasper   **Child Care: Some Nursing Perspectives**   1 870065 23 9
In three sections, this book covers many pertinent issues that are associated with caring for babies, young children and adolescents, in hospital and community settings.

Horne   **Effective Communication**   1 870065 14 X
This book examines a wide range of communication topics, including counselling, confidentiality, group and team work, compliance and communicating with children.

Horne   **Patient Education Plus**   1 870065 11 5
This book helps to develop nurses' teaching roles, and covers an extensive range of clinical topics. Each chapter contains a useful handout which can be freely photocopied or adapted for use with clients.

Horne   **Practice Check!**   1 870065 10 7
Each Practice Check presents a brief description of situations which may arise in practice together with open-ended questions and discussion to enable problems to be explored and effective solutions to be found.

Horne   **Staff Nurse's Survival Guide**   1 87 0065 13 1
Relevant to recently qualified and experienced nurses working in all healthcare settings, this brings together chapters on a wide range of clinical and non-clinical issues in patient care.

Horne   **Ward Sister's Survival Guide**   1 870065 12 3
This book is essential reading and a valuable reference for all nurses with direct clinical management responsibility.

Contents

Introduction

Focus on nursing skills

The Resource Management Initiative was launched in 1986 and gained increasing prominence by January 1989 in *Working for Patients* (HMSO, 1989) which stressed that the key to successful management of the NHS was good management of people. Although *Working for Patients* acknowledged that medically qualified consultants must be involved in the management of hospitals and given responsibility for the use of resources, it also acknowledged that nurses represent the largest professional group in the NHS, and that nurses must be afforded wider opportunities to make better use of their professional skills. As part of the Resource Management Initiative, local managers, including nurse managers, would be expected to identify the best use of professional skills, with the strong suggestion that a re-appraisal of traditional practices and patterns of care delivery would be a useful starting point.

Information generation and sharing

The ambitious timetable in *Working for Patients* reflected Government commitment in 1989 to the introduction of modern information systems to support both clinical and operational functions in hospitals. However, during 1990, it became apparent that this timescale was becoming increasingly impossible to achieve.

The Resource Management Initiative can only succeed if there are substantial reserves of cash to invest in information technology and training for staff to use technology to ease the reforms into place. Health Authorities and Provider Units still lack some of the information and expertise needed to run the contractual style new NHS. Information technology alone will not solve professional problems, information technology can by definition only manipulate data into information. There will always be a requirement for nurse managers of sufficient calibre to interpret the information and take decisions.

The question here is how should nursing information be utilised and decisions taken about nursing resources. Within the new contractual framework, such decisions will at last be explicit, since service agreements which form the basis for contracts must stipulate the amount of activity, the quality standards and the costs of treatment. Ward nurses must know the quality standards for their areas, and if nursing resources do not permit them to reach those quality standards, they are on a much sounder footing to draw attention to the fact.

It was recognised in *Working For Patients* that managers and professional staff required better information if they were to make the best uses of resources that were available to them. The Resource

Management Initiative is intended to provide a means of obtaining integrated, patient-based data which can be used to link information about the clinical needs of patients, the cost of treatment and the outcomes of such treatment to form a sound basis for clinical audit and quality assurance.

Cultural changes   The Resource Management Initiative is concerned with costs, technology and culture. Technology must provide a rapid, accurate, accessible and secure means of obtaining and integrating patient-based information about costs, and outcomes of treatment but the culture of the organisation must also change to become an information sharing culture, rather than an 'information is power' culture. The philosophy of multidisciplinary care for patients is familiar, yet in practice professional tribalism remains a dominant culture. Clinical directorates should underpin the shift to multidisciplinary care for patients with access to a shared information base.

Adopting the right strategy

The cultural changes in the NHS are long overdue. Nurses are the largest professional group in the NHS and should be leading the changes to pro-active management, rather than cling to re-active management. The way forward is well signposted by the targets identified in *Strategy For Nursing* (DOH, 1989). Nurses have a wealth of management expertise to offer but they must adopt the right strategy which cannot be based on crisis cost containment, but must focus on the differential contribution that nursing skills can make to desired patient outcomes.

References
DOH (1989) *A Strategy for Nursing: A Report of the Steering Committee. Department of Health Nursing Division, London.*
HMSO (1989) *Working for Patients.* HMSO, London.

Monica Duncan.
July, 1991.

Implementing Resource Management

1

Organisational changes and development issues

Lynn M. Dunne, MA, RGN, RCNT
Quality Assurance Adviser, Richmond, Twickenham and Roehampton Health Authority

In order to consider the organisational changes and development issues surrounding resource management properly, it is necessary to review the founding principles and values of the NHS.

Founding principles and values

The founding principles and values of the NHS were set out in the White Paper *A National Health Service* published by the British Government in February 1944 and are summarised as follows:

"The Government have announced that they intend to establish a comprehensive health service for everyone in this country. They want to ensure that in future:
1. Every man, woman and child can rely on getting all the advice, treatment and care which they may need in matters of personal health;
2. That what they get shall be the best medical and other facilities available.
3. That their getting these shall not depend on whether they can pay for them, or on any other factor irrelevant to the real need – the real need being to bring the country's full resources to bear upon reducing ill health and promoting good health in all its citizens."
4. The personal relationship between the patient and the doctor is preserved. "Throughout the Service must be based on the personal relationship of doctor and patient."
5. The danger of increased bureaucracy is avoided. "There is a certain danger in making personal health the subject of a national health service at all. It is the danger of over organisation, of letting the machine designed to ensure a better service itself stifle the chance of getting one."
6. Personal and professional freedom for the patient and doctor are preserved. "Nor should there be any compulsion into the Service, either for the patient or the doctor. The basis must be that the new service will be there for everyone that wants it but if anyone prefers not to use it, or likes to make private arrangements outside the Service, he must be at liberty to do so. Similarly, if any medical practitioner prefers not to take part in the new service and to rely wholly on private work, he must also

be at liberty to do so."

But if those were the values the reality was somewhat different. The whole concept of the NHS was based on Beveridge's theory that there was a fixed pool of ill health that would rapidly diminish, together with the costs of running the health service, as people were cured and the health of the population improved (leaving the service free to concentrate on the less costly aspects of health education and preventative medicine). The discovery and use of vaccines and antibiotics, the virtual elimination of Tuberculosis, improved anaesthetics and asepsis together with other dramatic advances in medical knowledge and technology significantly increased the life expectancy of the population and the incidence of chronic disease. These developments, which were not foreseen by Beveridge, have made the NHS in a sense a victim of its own success, with demand continually outstripping resources and therefore always requiring more funding.

I submit that the objective, to avoid increased bureaucracy, is incompatible with a centrally financed and controlled health service, given that the system must be governed by a vast set of fixed rules to ensure fairness and impartiality, particularly when the resources to be allocated are to be redistributed amongst those from whom funding was collected.

All these factors have had a catastrophic impact on the funding of healthcare and the management of resources and we should perhaps not be too surprised that a NHS based on the thinking of the 1940s should find itself in difficulties in the 1990s. Which brings us to the present situation and proposed reforms.

Organisational changes

It is important at the outset not to confuse resource management with the Government's proposed reforms of the health service and remember that resource management preceded *Working for Patients* by approximately three years. Resource management is nevertheless, with its emphasis on efficiency and economy, an integral part of the NHS reforms.

Next we need to consider what is the current thinking on organisational changes and developments necessary to achieve the optimal management of resources in today's NHS.

Establishing effective units   It could be argued that many of the problems encountered in running the NHS stem from the fact that those who deliver care to patients have had to-date no responsibility or accountability for the use of resources in discharging that function. Conversely those responsible for the management of resources have little appreciation of the issues involved in delivering a service to patients. Resource management aims to create effective links and communication between management and clinical staff through the use of management structures and processes to overcome this problem (Figure 1).

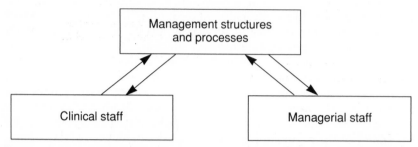

Figure 1. Communication links being formed between management and clinical staff.

Efficiency and effectiveness   Resource management also addresses what is now recognised as two separate production functions in the delivery of health care, namely efficiency and effectiveness. Traditionally efforts to improve the performance of the health service have concentrated on efficiency measures, eg, the efficient production of services such as nursing care, catering, laboratory tests etc or to put it more simply doing things right.

Resource management also considers the important aspect of effectiveness which is concerned with the prescribing of specific orders by the clinician/independent practitioner and is unique to health care or to put it more simply doing the right things. Successful resource management is an optimal combination of both efficiency and effectiveness.

Clinical Directorates   The organisational structure proposed for the implementation of resource management at grassroots level is the Clinical Directorate Model. Clinical Directorates (Figure 2) would

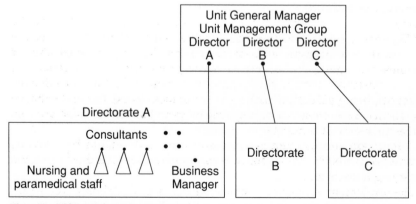

Figure 2. Clinical Directorate Model.

replace the present traditional management structure of Medical Executive Committee and Heads of Department/Service (Figure 3).

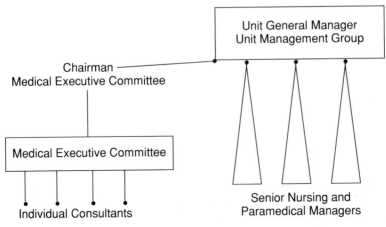

Figure 3. *Traditional model.*

Clinical Directorates are also being asked to produce a Business Plan for each Directorate that considers the following. issues:
1. Direction – where are we going?
2. Internal analysis – how are we doing?
3. External analysis – what are our competitors doing?
4. Making and monitoring progress – how do we know we are getting there?
(Peat, Marwick and McLintock, 1990)
    The important point to be made in all this is that we are not just being asked to put a new system in (as so often happened before). This time we are also being asked to adopt a new thinking and implement changes that will fundamentally affect the running of the NHS.

Development issues
There are many individuals who are worried about the notion of the NHS becoming more business like. In the end what matters is not the process of becoming more business like but the issue of what kind of business we want to be, ie, a commercial profit orientated organisation or a cooperative with savings, generated from efficient and effective practices, being ploughed back into the business to expand and enhance the service for the users and potential users of the service (who are also the main source of funding).
    If resource management is successful the result should be a leaner, more effective NHS that is more customer orientated. But there are some worrying aspects too.
    The implementation of the Clinical Directorate Model may well result in the loss of a professional structure for nursing (and other professional

groups) above Directorate level unless moves are made locally to protect it. Loss of the professional nursing structure raises concerns relating to leadership, quality assurance and professional development issues. Also within the Directorate, unless specifically agreed locally, there is no requirement that the nurse manager necessarily be a nurse. Whilst this is in keeping with the principles of general management, the attractions of running these large budgets must be matched with the necessary skills and an understanding of the relevant nursing issues if nursing is to survive unscathed.

There are also concerns for Community Services. Will Community Services become Directorates in their own right or will they be carved up between the Acute Services Directorates? Community Services units can be viewed if you will as the honest brokers of health care whose main aim is to keep the individual patient out of hospital and in the community where he/she belongs. If Community Services get swallowed up by the Acute Unit, then potentially so does the honest broker, which is bad news for patients and taxpayers alike as inpatient hospital-based care is more costly than home-based community care.

Clarity of vision

Lastly, resource management by itself is not enough. Unless the all important link between cost, quality and outcome are made a danger exists that patients, instead of resource management, will be used merely as means and not as ends in themselves. The all important link is mission – having a clearly stated concept of role and function. Or to paraphrase "what we are here to do" and "the way we want to do things around here", for it is here that the organisation can be clear about means and ends. In short, there is no ethical problem with resource management – in contrast with the internal market and the NHS. Indeed becoming more efficient and eliminating waste of scarce and precious resources is morally desirable, provided our actions are always determined with reference to respect for the autonomy of individuals, beneficence and equity.

References

Brunel University (1989 Resource Management: Process and Progress. Brunel University, London.

HMSO (1989) Working for Patients. HMSO, London.

Peat Marwick McLintock (1989) Review of the United Kingdom Central Council and the four National Boards for Nursing, Midwifery and Health Visiting. Department of Health, London.

2

Resource management: an overview

Jo Wilson, RGN, RM, RSCN, BSc (Hons), PG Dip Strategy and Resource Management
Regional Project Nurse, Resource Management, Northern Regional Health Authority

The impact of resource management on the nursing professions has meant that the nurses' role has become strengthened, making them totally responsible for all services and quality of care to their patients and clients.

The four key elements of resource management are:
- Improved quality of care.
- Involvement in management by those staff, such as nurses, doctors, and paramedics, whose decisions directly commit resources to patient treatment and care.
- Improved information.
- Effective control of resources.

Accessing information

The term 'resource management' refers to the information needed to control, measure and manage the resources needed and supplied for patient care. The change has been in providing clinical nurses with this vital information to aid their clinical and managerial responsibility and decision-making. The development of skills in reading, analysing and intepretating information is crucial in order to fulfil this managerial and clinical role. Professional decisions over resources need to be made by practising nurses as near to the bedside as possible. Research-based practice relies on the nurse's decision to identify individual patient needs.

The aim of the Resource Management Initiative was to help managers, health authorities, and others with a practical interest in the better use of the NHS resources, to make more informed judgements on the development of financial systems for their organisation. The information will allow doctors, nurses and other health care professionals within their units of control to review the mix of services and to rebalance them within existing resources.

Tracking resources related to patient care

With the development of a case mix database, all the data related to one patient can be stored in one file. These files are the feeder systems which will enable information related to nursing, physiotherapy, pathology, pharmacy, radiology, medical physics, finance, theatres, ECG, dietetics, etc to be passed across, making it possible to track a patient during his entire stay in hospital.

When the patient enters the hospital he will be allocated a hospital identification number, consultant and ward; the key piece of information is his identification number which will be the link with all the other systems. Once he arrives on a ward he will be assessed and put into a dependency group, the appropriate amount of nursing time will be allocated and this will be repeated each day during his stay. Each time he has a blood test, X-ray etc, these will be allocated to his identification number in the same way.

A global picture is then obtained of all the resources used for the patient during his entire stay. Costings can them be applied to the feeder systems. In addition the patient's diagnosis and procedures are coded to be able to compare similar cases.

Two coding systems can be used, one is the Operational Procedure Code System 4th series. This codes all operations and procedures the patient has during his stay. The other coding system is the International Code of Diseases ICD 9CM 9th series, which has clinical modifications to reflect the magnitude of diseases. This records the patient's primary diagnosis and up to five secondary diagnoses. As a result of both these coding systems the patient will be allocated to a Diagnostic Related Group (DRG). These diagnostic related groupings are taken from the USA and have their limitations in the UK. They are currently being adopted to reflect the magnitude of care under each of them. In this way the costs of cases in the same groupings can be compared.

With more effective provision and use of comparative health service indicators, the capability to assess efficiency, effectiveness and value for money will improve and can become increasingly related to establishing guidelines for good practice. Cases coming outside the normal patterns within the diagnostic related groupings can be examined to identify the reasons, such as poor home circumstances, lengthening stay in hospital or a more speedy recovery than was anticipated.

Nurse Management Information System

One of the key issues in implementing resource management is to have a Nurse Management Information System (NMIS) which will cover all nursing requirements but will be as simple as possible for staff to use to its full advantage.

Requirements The requirements of a Nurse Management Information System are:
- To provide information to allow more efficient management and utilisation of resources.

- To facilitate the assessment of the quality and effectiveness of the treatment and care provided to patients and clients.
- To provide individual patient costs.
- To provide direct operational benefits to staff by replacing current time-consuming manual systems and giving them the required information and control to organise their services.

The elements of any Nurse Management Information System centres around three areas which are a *workload measure, the rostering of staff* by grade and skill mix to give a good quality of care, and *care planning* as a mechanism to record, monitor and audit the level and quality of care (See Figure 1). These elements either individually or all together can

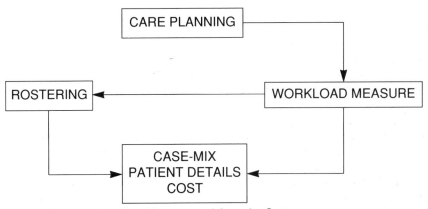

Figure 1. Elements of a Nurse Management Information System

provide case-mix details for individual patient costing. Nursing is one of the main feeder systems into resource management. An efficient nursing system should interface with the Patient Administration System (PAS), which is the medical records with the patients' biographical details and hospital number, and the Integrated Personnel System (IPS), which contains the staff details on grades and skills, and connects with the Finance department, which has the payroll cost details (See Figure 2). This saves duplication of information and valuable nursing time which can be better directed to patient care.

Uses   The uses of Nurse Management Information Systems are:
1. Setting nurse establishments.
2. Rostering indications using workload measure.
3. Enabling the Ward Sister and nursing staff to formally plan a nursing strategy for the ward.
4. Enabling nursing audit and standard setting.
5. Providing objectives for staff individual performance review.
6. Providing case-mix information and nurse/patient costings.

The Nurse Management Information System indicates the importance of

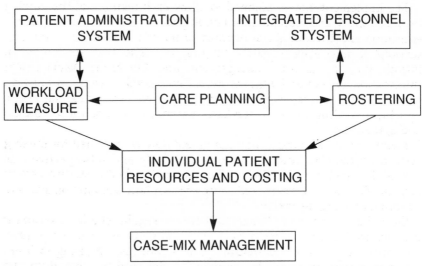

Figure 2. An efficient Nurse Management Information System interfaces with the Patient Administration System and the Integrated Personnel System.

nursing and its pivotal role in co-ordination and continuity of patient care. It aids management of the ward, but does not replace it, it informs nurses of all the choices they have to make. The basic approach is openness in providing information, support, training and education to nursing staff and other interested parties. It is timed to suit the needs of the ward and needs widespread consultation in implementation.

Implementing the system

All three, or two, or only one element of the Nurse Management Information System can be implemented on a ward. At Freeman Hospital we started with implementing a workload measure, because we felt it would lead to better care planning and rostering of nursing staff, which could be computerised at a later date. After consultation, Criteria for Care was chosen as it appeared to be the best system to suit the needs and culture of the District Health Authority.

The Nurse Management Information System we then developed is based on the use of Criteria for Care and Monitor. Criteria for Care is a manpower planning method which enables the amount of nursing time and skills required to meet the needs of a variety of different patient groups to be assessed and provides a desired standard of care. Monitor is based upon a study which assesses the quality of care, giving a patient and ward-centred quality indicator of care and identifying areas for quality improvements. The system looks at the demand for nursing care using the classification (based on nursing care plans and implemented care) which gives the workload index, the supply of nursing staff in nurse hours to give the care and the quality of care delivered.

The implementation is planned to allow each member of the nursing team to receive and read an information pack at least two weeks prior to education and training. Each member of nursing staff has two training sessions lasting approximately 90 minutes. The first session is an introduction to resource management, and the Nurse Management Information System and all it involves. The second session is a practical session where nursing staff bring along patient care plans and assess patients according to the dependency criteria, with time for discussion and agreement.

Following the training a commencement date is identified for nursing staff to do the classification, both prospectively and retrospectively as part of the lunch-time handover. The trainer attends the handover every day for the first two weeks and comments on how the nursing staff are adapting to using the system.

Once the system is implemented there are regular checks to ensure it is being used in a reliable and valid way, and that the dependency levels are reflected within the individual patient care plan. Nursing staff are taught how to calculate the workload index and to give them the nursing hours required to give the desired level of care. They can then compare these to the nursing hours available from the duty roster. Once computer training is complete, this is done automatically in seconds, but having performed the calculation manually aids staff understanding.

It takes a fair amount of work to get the system up and running on a ward but once the system has been developed it does have benefits to the ward staff.

Changes and benefits

As a result of effectively using the Nurse Management Information System and having observational studies performed, different wards have changed practices in many ways. Some of these are outlined to show how the Ward Sister can make the most efficient and effective use of her nursing resources to their fullest potential. Other changes are developing through a structural approach to change to ensure it is functional, measured and evaluated.

Changes in the patient's day By looking at what is done for the patient when and how, the idea is to make things as normal for the patient as possible. Waking patients before 0700 hours in order to accomplish ward routine before the day staff arrives has stopped. Nursing care is given on a 24 hour basis and planned according to the patient's individual needs. Nurses are challenging historical routines and practices, such as frequency in recording vital signs, when daily observations should be undertaken, when drug rounds should occur leading to less structured ward routines.

24 hour rostering With introducing 24 hour rostering, this has enabled full control over the 24 hour period, with full accountability when trying to match the demands of patients with the supply of nursing staff. This includes internal rotation to allow better continuity of care while giving an appreciation of the different pressures over the 24 hour day.

Flexible rostering   With flexible rostering this enables nursing staff to alter their duty patterns according to the assessed needs of the patients. This obviously needed much discussion and overall staff agreement for it to work effectively. It is now operating on surgical, medical and rheumatology wards. It may not work on all wards and therefore needs to be seen as useful to the staff themselves and not forced upon them. It allows nurses to be on duty when the patients need them, rather than having fixed duty patterns with some unnecessary staff overlaps.

In practice on the days where supply exceeds demand, nurses take time owing and are prepared to work extra when the ward is busy. Some weeks nurses work extra and take time back when it is quieter, over a four week period the staff clear any surplus or deficits. The ward therefore becomes much more self-sufficient and the nurses cater for the peaks and troughs of activity. It is better for patient care as nursing staff who know the patients are there when required, instead of relying on borrowed or bank staff.

Concentrated direct care by the trained staff   By examining the associated work, some of which can be considered non-nursing duties, more direct care is being undertaken by the trained nurses. More of the stock and supplies and housekeeping tasks are being undertaken by the auxiliaries and support workers. Also more associated work is being done overnight when patients are sleeping, and preparatory work can be undertaken to allow more staff time with the patients when they are awake.

Introduction of new duties times   Some wards have introduced a new duty time of either 1000–1800 hours or 1100–1900 hours to allow nursing staff to be on duty for busier times before patients' lunch and supper. Going off later has advantages for surgical wards especially when theatre patients need concentrated care in the immediate postoperative period.

Unit/ward admission policies   Unit and ward admission policies are being considered with empty beds not being the sole reason for admitting patients to the ward. It would be more useful to encourage medical staff to consult the workload information and the nursing staff hours available. This would ensure patients receive better quality care and would limit boarding out of patients from ward to ward. Many advantages of this policy could be envisaged for better care and continuity of care.

Better care planning　As a result of using the dependency Nurse Management Information System as an integral part of the nursing process, patients' care plans have become much more specific. Nursing staff find assessment and goal setting easier, because they are planning ahead and predicting the dependency level with the patient. Better evaluation has resulted due to recording retrospectively the dependency levels. The care plans should become so specific that when auditing them the dependency level of the patient is evident.

Primary nursing and team nursing　Better organised delivery of nursing care through primary nursing and team nursing gives more continuity of care and better prediction of patient care. This leads to more concentrated care by individual nurses and better continuity of care for patients.

Quality issues　The setting of ward objective around Monitor resulted in the highlighting of areas where quality can be improved. By developing staff awareness of quality, it identifies areas of excellence or deficit, and helps them to make better use of the nursing process and documentation of nursing care. Standard setting and quality audit of care plans takes place regularly by the Ward Sister and nursing staff.

Giving good quality patient care

Resource management is here to aid the professional nurse to provide the information, power and control necessary to give the best service to patients. It does not replace the human resources and must be influenced by professional judgement each step of the way. All the computerised systems which are available giving workload measures, typed care plans and rostering of staff with costs, are all singing and dancing coloured graphs and systems. They are here to aid and help the professional nurse in the control of resources and decision-making, but they will never replace the nurse and her professional judgement. They are here to help in the management of the ward, saving valuable trained staff time which can be better directed to giving good quality patient care.

3

What is resource management?

Shirley Williams, RGN, RHV
Director of Nursing Services (Community Services), Oxford H.A. Formerly Director of Nursing Services, Radcliffe Infirmary, Oxford

A major complaint voiced by nurses is that they have an ever increasing workload without any commensurate increase in staffing. As a result they are unable to provide what they consider to be an acceptable standard of care. There is considerable evidence to support the claim that workload has risen both in volume and intensity.

- Shorter length of stay has resulted in a rise in the dependency of those patients who are in hospital.
- Quicker throughput may mean the patient due for admission arrives before the patient occupying his or her prospective bed has been discharged. This means the nurses have more patients than beds (and staffing establishments are traditionally set on bed numbers).
- Increasingly sophisticated medical procedures often require added nursing support.

Not surprisingly, the increase in the number of patients treated has resulted in a marked rise in expenditure, particularly in non-staff items such as drugs, X-rays and prosthesis. This has generated considerable alarm in government circles.

Cash limits

In an attempt to control what appeared to be runaway expenditure, 'cash limits' were introduced whereby district health authorities were instructed to ensure they contained their spending within the funds they were allocated. Many health authorities simply passed this directive down the line, and in some cases budget holders found themselves being reprimanded for 'overspending' when they had no idea what money they had been allocated, nor what they were expected to achieve with it.

As a result of cash limits, hospitals found themselves between a pincer movement. On the one hand they were under pressure from the Department to maximise use of their resources, with particular reference to such things as theatre time, while on the other hand they were being reprimanded for expenditure above that which had been allocated by the department, but which had been incurred as a result of the very increase in efficiency which the hospital had been instructed to undertake. The NHS enquiry tried to address this dilemma, and Griffiths said it was necessary for "each unit to develop management budgets which involve clinicians and relate workload and service objectives to financial and manpower allocations".

There was, however, a major obstacle preventing the achievement of Griffiths' aim. The NHS had no idea of the cost of individual components of treatment and care. Previously it had not been deemed necessary to have a pricing policy, since there had been no requirement to 'bill' a patient. However, if Griffiths' ideas were to be realised it would be essential to identify how money was being spent; and work has been going on in this area in a number of pilot sites, on a system of *providing* management information known as resource management. *is*

The resource management initiative involves the following:

- Agreeing clear objectives with doctors, nurses and other hospital managers.
- Agreeing with them budgets related to their workload and objectives.
- Giving them greater control over the day-to-day use of resources.
- Providing better information on the actual cost of clinical activity and services used by clinicians and patients.
- Holding budget-holders accountable for their performance.
- Reviewing outcome.

The resource management system will, where these basic principles are applied to a specialty or clinical service, base the information on an individual patient episode, linking the costs to discharge diagnosis, and perhaps ultimately a diagnostic group. Doctors and nurses can then not only understand the potential of their overall budgets to manage their service, but the effects their case-mix has on this.

Thus, with resource management we move from attempting to cope with an unplanned, demand-led workload within a cash limited financial allocation to a position where there is agreement about the amount of work which can be accomplished within available resources. It is imperative that nurses play an assertive proactive role in agreeing workload related budgets, since it is us and only us who can make the necessary statements about what constitutes nursing workload. The way in which we nurses approach this will be determined by our own understanding of the nature of nursing work.

What is nursing?

If we believe nursing consists of the execution of a series of largely predetermined tasks, we are likely to think it appropriate to deploy any nurse to carry out any task in any area. With such a philosophy it is possible to separate the responsibility for the proficient completion of the task from authority over the resources to carry them out. This position is clearly reflected in traditional nurse management arrangements, where ward sisters are held responsible for standards of care on their wards, but have minimal control over the composition of their establishment or deployment of their staff. Their day duty plans can be overridden by the nursing officer or duty nurse who has authority to redeploy their staff; and their responsibility for and authority over night duty is often either tenuous or a subject of outright hostility between themselves and the night sister. In a traditional system the duty nurse, both on day duty and at night, has resources of her own in the shape of a pool or team, which she deploys on a shift by shift basis at her own discretion.

In a task orientated hospital, the approach to resource management would be to devise a system where all tasks were identified and timed and all nursing resources were controlled centrally so that they could be deployed on a shift by shift basis in response to the predicted task-constituted workload and then be 'costed' at patient level. Many hospitals are taking this approach and indeed the production of computerised nurse deployment systems to support them is a new growth industry.

So where should a ward sister start when implementing a resource management system? A report from the Department of Health's Nursing Division (1988) reviewed the issues. It is first helpful to draw up three component functions that could make up a ward based management information system – the functions are:

- workload assessment;
- ward nurse tracking (recording past, present and planned future shift and work patterns of individual staff);
- care planning support.

Workload assessment

Systematic methods of assessing the demand for nurse manpower date back to the late 1950s. A vast amount has been written in the UK and America dealing with the various issues arising in this area of nursing demand, with conflicting claims as to the which is the best approach. It is vital to have some understanding of these issues before designing a resource management system.

Clearly, to decide how many nurses should be on a particular ward at a particular time is not simply a question of measurement – some judgement is also necessary, but existing approaches can vary a great deal in the level of detail they require. Some simply focus on 'nursing tasks', while others go into more detail, classifying patients into dependency groups. Greater complexity and detail does not necessarily bring greater accuracy, however. Schroeder at al (1984), in a trial between two systems found an easy to establish and simple to operate one gave essentially the same results as a more cumbersome task orientated system. They recommended that nurses avoid adopting expensive, detailed task orientated staffing tools, and depend on systems developed in-house by their own nursing staff, which the staff are happy using. This view has also been endorsed by the NHS Management Board (Peach, 1987).

The question of whether the resource management systems should be used to formulate nursing process care plans is a contentious one. It is unlikely that nurses would willingly accept the idea that workload derived task specifications could or should play a role in care planning. Part of the philosophy of individualised care planning is to move away from the mechanical, task-based approach to patient care. It is probably wise, therefore, to keep the care planning process separate from the resource management system, otherwise the system may end up fulfilling neither of the functions for which it is intended. However, since nursing workload is generated by a patient's need for care, the level of nursing resource required will be reflected in his care plan. The amount of care he actually receives will be determined by a combination of the level of total nursing resources available and the priority of his needs against those of other patients who have a call on the same resources. Whilst not strictly part of resource management, it is important to identify any discrepancy between care needed and care received if we are to include the added dimension of quality.

Use of computers

Computers can be useful tools in resource management, and their use can have a number of advantages. Information retrieval is quick and easy, and all the information is easily stored without taking up precious space. However, individual ward sisters need to ask whether using a computer will be better for them than a preprinted form to be completed by hand. When nurses are busy and documentation is not seen as a priority, it is just as easy to produce misleading and incomplete computer records as it is hand written ones, so computers should not be seen as a way of imposing a discipline which guards against this. If they are to be used, it should be because the ward sister (and the rest of the staff) feel computerisation will genuinely allow them to operate their resource management system more efficiently and effectively.

Government commitment

The recent White Paper (DoH, 1989) makes it clear the Government is committed to the expansion of the resource management initiative. It is imperative that nurses ensure the opportunities it affords are used for the benefit of patient care, and that the exercise does not merely become a costing mechanism to help the accountants ensure that 'the money follows the patient'.

It is important that hospitals understand the implications of introducing resource management. Merely introducing modern information systems to record clinical and operational activities will achieve nothing except perhaps lots of pretty pie charts. At whatever level a hospital decides it is best to turn its clinical services – involving doctors, nurses and other professionals – it must be based on the principle that the people responsible for care need to be given clear areas of responsibility. This must be supported by an agreed budget which is related to a level and quality of service that can be reasonably be provided within the funds available.

An appropriate management philosophy – and a proper structure within the unit to support it – is an essential prerequisite for the successful introduction of resource management.

References

DoH (1988) *The Resource Management Initiative and Ward Nursing Management Information Systems.* DoH Nursing Division and Operational Research Services, London.

DoH (1989) *Working for Patients.* HMSO, London.

Peach, L. (1987) Nurse manpower planning. Letter to regional and district general managers. Ref DA (87)**12**.

Schroeder, R.E., Rhodes, A., Shields, R.E. (1984) Nurse acuity services: CASH vs GRASP (a determination of nurse staff requirements). *Journal of Nursing Administration, 21, 2, 72-77.*

4

Making resource management work

Jan Chalmers, RGN
Theatre Service Manager, Radcliffe Infirmary, Oxford

Resource management was implemented at the Radcliffe Infirmary based on our belief in the value of professional judgment and the importance of building teams to facilitate a high standard of individualised patient care. We believe decisions regarding patient care and the authority over resources to provide that care should be made as near to the bedside as possible.

The changes in our nursing structure described in this chapter were made in line with this philosophy. We moved from a task orientated approach to what we believe to be the much firmer ground of professional practice.

Professional practice is based on the nurse's responsibility to identify individual patient needs. The example used to illustrate this in a recent Nurses and Midwives Advisory Council's circular suggests the question ceases to be "How quickly can I take the temperature of all my patients?" and becomes, "Which patient's temperature do I need to monitor and how frequently?" Acceptance of professional practice has a profound effect on the way nursing is managed, particularly in the choice of level at which responsibility and authority for decision making is placed.

Key role of ward sisters

Ward sisters   At the Radcliffe Infirmary, each ward has one sister or charge nurse who works primarily on day duty with a 24-hour, 365-day-a-year responsibility for the quality of nursing on the ward. This also involves occasional night duty when required.

Ward sisters have 'ownership' of non-staff expenditure and the staffing resources for the ward and the authority to decide how nursing staff on the ward will be deployed and what the skill mix will be (see Table 1). In addition, they negotiate an agreed workload for the ward with medical staff, so controlling non-emergency admissions to the ward.

Senior ward sisters   Wards are grouped together in specialty units, for example elderly care, neurosurgery etc. The sister (or charge nurse) in charge of one of the wards within a particular specialty unit is responsible

```
REPORT NUMBER  ORG/0042SCS                    OXFORD REGIONS BUSINESS INFORMATION SYSTEMS (ORBIS)                      PAGE:        84
MR:   CV RI - OPTHALMOLOGY                         BUDGET MANAGER'S SUBJECTIVE REPORT :                               DATE:  10/01/91
09 MONTHS ENDING 31/12/90                            COST CENTRE 20970 THEATRES - OEH                                 TIME:  08:49:55

COMMENTS:
```

STAFFING CURRENT MONTH BUDGET WORKED WTE	CURRENT MONTH ACTUAL WORKED WTE	AVERAGE Y.T.D. ACTUAL WORKED WTE	CODE	SUBJECTIVE DESCRIPTION	ANNUAL BUDGET £	CURRENT MONTH BUDGET £	ACTUAL £	VARIANCE £	YEAR TO DATE BUDGET £	ACTUAL £	VARIANCE £	CF %
1.00	1.00	0.45	122505	GRADE G NURSE	19472	1623	1410	213-	14607	15354	747	5.1
1.00	1.00	0.81	123005	GRADE F NURSE	16804	1400	1159	241-	12600	12097	503-	4.0-
2.50	2.28	2.20	123505	GRADE E NURSE	33514	2792	2503	289-	25128	23131	1997-	7.9-
2.53	1.52	2.50	124005	GRADE D NURSE	18983	2646	1454	1192-	11040	21610	10570	95.7
2.39	0.44	0.20	124505	GRADE C NURSE	21852	1821	322	1499-	16389	1291	15098-	92.1-
0.00	0.00	0.00	156410	OPERAT DEPT AS BG	0	0	0	0	0	0	0	0.0
0.00	0.00	0.00	156415	OPER DEP ASS TRAI	0	0	113	113	0	391	391	0.0
9.42	**6.24**	**6.16**		**PAY TOTAL**	**110625**	**10282**	**6961**	**3321-**	**79764**	**73875**	**5889-**	**7.4-**
			301506	DRUGS-STORES ISSU	0	0	5	5	0	18	18	0.0
			310505	MEDICAL GASES	0	0	0	0	0	105	105	0.0
			311005	DRESSINGS-PURCHAS	0	0	0	0	0	20	20	0.0
			311006	DRESSING-STORE IS	0	0	766	766	0	1010	1010	0.0
			311503	MSSE-PURCHASES-DI	0	0	23	23	0	10375	10375	0.0
			311504	MSSE-PUR-NON DISP	0	0	0	0	0	503	503	0.0
			311510	MSSE-STORES ISSUE	0	0	197	197	0	1668	1668	0.0
			311565	OPTICAL EQUIPMENT	0	0	33	33	0	378	378	0.0
			311580	SURGICAL INST DIS	0	0	0	0	0	9650	9650	0.0
			311581	SURGICAL INST-GEN	0	0	0	0	0	1613	1613	0.0
			311582	SURG INST NON DIS	38300	3192	0	3192-	25536	0	25536-	100.0-
			311587	SURG INST-OPHTHAL	0	0	0	0	0	2833	2833	0.0
			311589	SURG INST-ORTHOPA	0	0	0	0	0	93	93	0.0
			311592	SUTURES	0	0	1310	1310	0	10949	10949	0.0
			311592	SYRINGES	0	0	22	22	0	22	22	0.0
			311740	LENS IMPLANTS	114860	9571	3137	6434-	76568	41750	34818-	45.5-
			311750	OTHER PROSTHESIS	0	0	0	0	0	246	246	0.0
			312045	PLIERS/INSTR.ORTH	0	0	443	443	0	443	443	0.0
			313045	MED EQUIP MAINTEN	0	0	0	0	0	69	69	0.0
			315100	PAT APPLI OPTICAL	0	0	78	78	0	78	78	0.0
			316005	LABORATORY OPTIFM	0	0	0	0	0	452	452	0.0
			316006	LAB EQ-STORES ISS	0	0	0	0	0	25	25	0.0
			322011	STAFF UNIFORMS SI	0	0	0	0	0	36	36	0.0
			322020	GLOVES-DISPOSABLE	0	0	383	383	0	383	383	0.0
			324506	BED&LINEN-DISP-SI	0	0	0	0	0	9	9	0.0
			330506	PRINT&STATION-SI	0	0	0	0	0	10	10	0.0
			332505	STAFF ADVERTISING	100	8	0	8-	64	0	64-	100.0-
			333005	TRAVELLING EXPENS	0	0	1	1	0	1	1	0.0
			333020	TRAVEL EXP-STANDA	0	0	98	98	0	164	164	0.0
			333030	TRAV EX-PASS MILE	0	0	1	1	0	1	1	0.0
			343072	TRANS.OF TRANSPLA	0	0	160	160	0	1075	1075	0.0
			385500	ALL OTHER EXPENDI	0	0	0	0	0	113	113	0.0
			391005	SER REC OTHER HA	0	0	160-	160-	0	0	0	0.0
				NON PAY TOTAL	**153260**	**12771**	**6496**	**6275-**	**102168**	**84093**	**18075-**	**17.7-**
9.42	**6.24**	**6.16**		**COST CENTRE TOTAL**	**263885**	**23053**	**13457**	**9596-**	**181932**	**157967**	**23965-**	**13.2-**

Table 1.

for coordinating the activities of the other sisters in the unit. Designated 'senior ward sister', they are assisted by a junior sister in their own ward.

Each senior sister is a member of the specialty team responsible for monitoring and planning work in the specialty unit. Other members of the team are the consultant, an administrator and an accountant. The specialty teams meet quarterly to review workload and expenditure

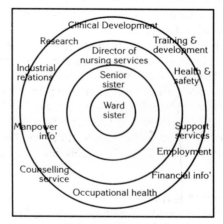

Figure 1. The ward sister is the centre of the devolution of authority to ward level.

under the chairmanship of the unit general manager. The senior sister also acts as the specialty unit's spokesperson, representing its interests either to the director of nursing services (DNS) or to other professional groups in the hospital. Senior sisters have direct assess to the DNS, to whom they are professionally and managerially accountable.

This access to the DNS means the conventional (and often non-clinical) role of nursing officer has been discontinued at the Radcliffe Infirmary. The responsibility and authority awarded to ward sisters has removed a tier of management which previously dealt with the central deployment of staff in the hospital. (See Figure 1). Traditional nursing officer posts (whose holders expected to directly influence clinical practice) were redesigned as support roles to facilitate the introduction of resource management.

Preparation and support of staff

The key to the successful implementation of resource management at ward level is the adequate preparation and ongoing support of ward sisters, who are responsible for the smooth working of the system.

By abolishing the nursing officer role and subsequently reorganising and redeploying nursing personnel within individual wards, we released resources for four new posts. Two clinical practice development nurses were appointed, and these are clinically involved with all wards in the hospital, helping them develop their clinical practice at whatever pace is appropriate for the nursing team involved. Clinical practice development nurses also organise workshops, undertake research and act as personal 'mentors' for individual nurses and ward teams.

The two other new posts were designed specifically to support organisational development and the introduction of resource management and it is to these posts that I and my colleague, Kate Woods were appointed. We were both expected to play a leading role in managing change, as well as providing professional and managerial support to all the ward sisters in the hospital.

These two posts provided professional and personal support to individuals and ward teams and were vital to the nursing system. Each has its own specific areas of expertise:

• Responsibility for organising and managing the devolution of the nursing budget to ward level, with ongoing responsibility for yearly budget setting, skill mix and recruitment issues and support and guidance for sisters in interpreting financial information.
• Responsibility for workload, quality tools and the development of trained staff.

Budget control at ward level

A knowledge of the resources currently available is a prerequisite for effective budgetary control at ward level. A first step was to help each ward sister identify the total size of her nursing establishment - a matter about which many ward sisters were unclear. After a nursing establishment for each ward was agreed upon, it was important to reassure the sisters that there could be no change to this without their approval.

After gaining the confidence of a particular ward sister in this way, we discussed whether or not the skill mix in the ward was fully suited to its patients' needs. It was evident that on some wards the mix was not ideal, either because of changes in medical practice or because of a failure to recruit appropriately trained nurses. On one ward, a senior ward sister was assisted by a total of only three whole time equivalent (WTE) trained nurses, and had seven nursing auxiliaries. After discussion, she changed the skill mix within her overall budget by appointing three additional trained nurses and redeploying five of the seven auxiliaries. This resulted in a new skill mix which was better suited to changed medical practices and her current nursing requirements.

A simple device which helped nurses assess the scope for modifying the skill mix within a fixed budget was a table showing how many hours of a particular grade equated (in salary cost terms) to how many hours of another grade (Table 2). Reference to the table showed, for example, that on average the salary of one Whole Time Equivalent (WTE) Grade

Payscales	A(<18)	A(>18)	B(18)	B(18+)	C	D	E	F	G	H	I
	1.00	1.00	1.00	1.00	1.00	1.00	1.00	1.00	1.00	1.00	1.00
A(<18)	1.00	1.26	1.31	1.45	1.70	1.94	2.22	2.55	2.91	3.23	3.56
A(>18)	.79	1.00	1.04	1.16	1.35	1.54	1.76	2.02	2.32	2.57	2.83
B(18)	.77	.96	1.00	1.11	1.30	1.48	1.70	1.95	2.23	2.47	2.72
B(18+)	.69	.87	.90	1.00	1.17	1.33	1.53	1.75	2.00	2.22	2.45
C	.59	.74	.77	.86	1.00	1.14	1.31	1.50	1.72	1.90	2.10
D	.52	.65	.67	.75	.88	1.00	1.15	1.32	1.50	1.67	1.84
E	.45	.57	.59	.65	.76	.87	1.00	1.15	1.31	1.45	1.60
F	.39	.49	.51	.57	.67	.76	.87	1.00	1.14	1.27	1.40
G	.34	.43	.45	.50	.58	.66	.76	.87	1.00	1.11	1.22
H	.31	.39	.40	.45	.53	.60	.69	.79	.90	1.00	1.10
I	.28	.35	.37	.41	.48	.54	.62	.72	.82	.91	1.00

Table 2. Whole time equivalent trade-off matrix for the clinical Grading Structure, calculated as cost based mean of all points of scale. The horizontal payscale reference shows the post to be traded at 1.00 W.T.E. The vertical payscale reference shows the different values that can be "bought".

A nursing auxiliary over 18 years of age is equivalent to 0.65 WTE of a Grade D staff nurse/enrolled nurse or 0.57 WTE of a Grade E staff nurse.

Using a fixed annual budget

Sisters are not held to account every month since the agreement is based on an estimated annual workload. This is important. Previously, if sisters had an establishment of 10 nurses, they would have been required to ensure this number was not exceeded, but they now have the authority to 'spend' the equivalent of 10 salaries over a full year and are encouraged to use their discretion over the way this is used. For example, one month a sister may have a vacancy but because none of her staff are on maternity or sick leave, the ward can function safely and satisfactorily. The following month she may theoretically have 10 nurses in post, but with one on maternity leave and several off sick she needs to 'buy' more nursing hours for her patients, either through overtime payments or by employing bank nurses. By doing this, the sister can provide nursing care for the same overall workload in each month by using only nine salaries during the first month and 11 salaries during the second.

There are many similar ways in which ward sisters can make flexible use of resources within a fixed annual budget. If, for example, over a period of several months they have been unable to recruit up to the full level of their establishment, they could use the money saved to buy a hoist to assist the depleted nursing team when lifting patients.

The ward sisters receive financial information every month to help them manage the resources for which they alone are responsible. This information gives details of budgeting and expenditure from the beginning of the year to date.

Consolidating the new role

If ward sisters are to fulfil their new role, it is essential that they are given adequate preparation to enable them to relate with other disciplines. The preparatory programme consisted of a negotiation skills workshop, a resource management module set up by the local polytechnic and a series of assertiveness sessions to develop their role in multidisciplinary teamwork and to gain increased personal confidence. With the help of these aids, staff were fully able to undertake their new roles brought about through the implementation of resource management.

Human Resources and Planning

5

Reaching the year 2000: manpower planning

Trevor Patchett, BA, AHSM, AIPM
Healthcare Partner, Price Waterhouse, London

Effective manpower planning is vital to the efficient running of the health service. Attention focused on this vital topic has increased since Price Waterhouse reported on the cost and manpower implications of Project 2000. An important reason for this interest and concern focuses on the issue of whether we will have the numbers of nurses required to provide the level of service planned for the coming years. Price Waterhouse have produced data to forecast the effect of the 'demographic timebomb' that lies in the reduction in the available number of 18 year olds and of the potential effects on manpower levels of the Project 2000 proposals.

What is manpower planning?

Manpower planning in its most basic definition is the balancing of the supply of and demand for labour for a given set of activities.

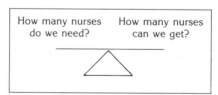

Figure 1. Balancing supply and demand.

If the two sides of Figure 1 are out of balance, the impact is felt directly in the clinical setting. The impact may take the shape of a lack of appropriately trained staff for a specific specialty at a particular time, or of a plethora of students or trained staff. In the past, attention has been paid to the question of "how many nurses do we need" (Telford, 1979; Mackley and Heslop, 1979; Cameron, 1979; Rhys Hern, 1979; Barr, 1964 and 1984), that is on demand modelling. But, as Figure 1 suggests, the need for staff must be balanced by the availability of staff, that is the *supply* of staff. Fundamental to the success of demand and supply manpower modelling is an information base which does not currently exist within the NHS. Two examples will highlight this:

Student service contribution   It is generally accepted that learners on basic nursing courses contribute to patients' care during the course of their training. It is also accepted that the extent of this service contribution varies both by course and by training school depending on the way particular courses are organised and on the extent to which certain clinical placements are supernumerary. In a lot of authorities student intakes have been cut either by failure to recruit or as a cost saving exercise. If authorities are not aware of the level of service contribution made by learners, how can they calculate the effect of the reduction in learner numbers on workload, or on the need for replacement qualified staff? Price Waterhouse's research showed that most authorities could not answer the question: What is the level of service contribution by course or by year of training?

Qualified staff wastage   Replacing qualified staff who leave the authority is the primary determinant of the number of learners to be taken into training. Yet many authorities are unable to quantify the rate of qualified staff wastage as they do not have data about where the staff go or why they leave.

The lack of such information makes effective manpower planning difficult, but if in the future we are to provide the type of service we wish, manpower plans have to be attempted in order to estimate the number of student nurses required at a time when the supply of 18 year olds is reducing.

Supply modelling

A supply model is a framework to identify the sources of and size of the supply of nursing staff. The key questions to be asked are:
- How many qualified staff do we need?
- How many qualified staff do we lose?
- Where do we get our qualified staff from?

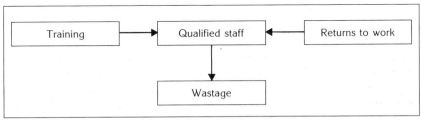

Figure 2. A simple supply model.

The questions enable us to construct a simple supply model as shown in Figure 2. However, Figure 2 is incomplete. Although the answers to the questions will identify how many qualified nurses need to be recruited and how many will be newly qualified it does not address the earlier question of how many students need to be recruited. Two further

questions must be asked:
- How many students leave training and when?
- How many students take their final exams and pass?

For a complete picture, additional questions should be asked about the numbers of unqualified staff, their retention rates and their wastage patterns. These provide the more comprehensive supply model that has been developed by Price Waterhouse for the NHS Nursing Workforce (Figure 3). The numbers in the diagram relate to 1990.

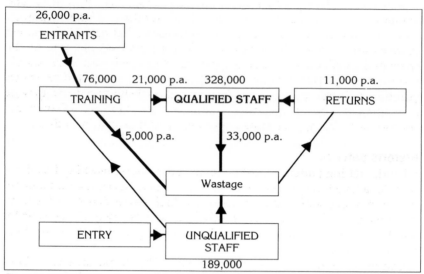

Figure 3. The NHS Nursing Workforce – simplified manpower model.

What does the model tell us?

The NHS loses 10 per cent of its qualified workforce each year, that is, 30,000 of the 300,000 qualified nurses in employment. Of this wastage only 30 per cent is made up by qualified staff returning. Yet these returning qualified staff are among the most cost-effective recruits to the workforce. Unfortunately, the emphasis, for example, in the southern part of England, has been on sending recruitment parties to Ireland and Scotland to fill the gap caused by falling school rolls, rather than on investigating the potential for enticing back to work already qualified staff who may live locally. The need to attract qualified nurses back to the profession not only makes economic sense but also is imperative if the number of qualified nurses is to be maintained in the event of a shortfall in recruitment to basic training. It is expected that women should have breaks in their career, but what should not be expected is the total loss of two thirds of those leaving the profession. 'Return to nursing' courses should be available to enable nurses who wish to return to refresh their skills and self-confidence. Authorities should not claim shortages of trained staff for specialist clinical areas while not offering Back to Nursing courses. The model points clearly to the need to address the problem of high wastage and low return to the profession.

The model shows 27,000 entrants to training: the great majority of these are females with between five 'O' levels and two 'A' levels going into first level training. Male and mature entrants are very small groups: consideration must be given to attracting greater numbers from these two groups into training and thus alleviating the dramatic effect of the reduction in the number of 18 year old females.

Given the current constraints on the availability of money and manpower there is need for a much closer scrutiny of staff resources. Obviously not every contingency can be foreseen, but better information systems and communications can reduce the impact of some of the changes. In addition, the nursing appraisal scheme, where it exists, should produce valuable information about the career intentions and prospects of individual staff. In an area of known national shortage there may be a requirement for exceptional action, such as provision of housing, sponsored training, accelerated promotion or financial incentives.

Historic patterns

Historic staffing patterns must be reviewed. London teaching hospitals, have for a long time prided themselves on employing a minimum number of non-nursing staff, with a consequent high dependence on learners. They have also had a history of only retaining newly qualified staff for short periods. Innovative methods of solving this high intake/high wastage problem must be explored.

Can the dependence on students remain? The simple answer is "no". Project 2000, which is now being widely implemented, will dramatically reduce the student contribution, while at the same time entrants to training will become more difficult to attract. Hence a reappraisal is needed and quickly. If both the volume and quality of service are to be maintained an examination must be undertaken on the:

- parameters of nursing;
- skill mix;
- factors affecting the retention of staff.

The manpower planning model that has been described relates primarily to forward and strategic planning. In addition to getting the overall numbers right, the profession has to address the problem of getting the right staff to the right place at the right time. At the operational/clinical level other planning systems are required based on how much activity takes place, when and how. Such planning systems lead to a consideration of the deployment of staff at ward or community locality level.

At a local level

To achieve equity at local level, it will be necessary to supply the information to enable the demand and supply equation to be balanced within the parameters of an agreed quality of service. Planned changes in workload should be identified as far in advance as possible and the manpower implications quantified. Unplanned changes in workload should be picked up on a day to day basis by a workload measurement system, and translated into a staffing requirement.

For the longer term, the supply side of the manpower equation has to be calculated from a model such as that shown in Figure 3, used in conjunction with a demand model. Information from the appraisal system and feedback from managers continually tests the sensitivities of staffing in key areas. Only by clinical nurses working with manpower planners, using the tools of demand and supply modelling, can we attempt to get the right staff in the right place at the right time.

References
Barr, A. (1964) Measuring nursing care. In: McLachlan, G. (Ed) *Problems and progress in Medical Care*. Nuffield Provincial Hospitals Trust, London.
Barr, A. (1984) Hospital nursing establishments and cost. *Hospital and Health Service Review*, **80**, 1,31-37.
Cameron, J. (1979) The Aberdeen Formula: revision of nursing workload per patient as a basis for staffing. *Nursing Times*, Occasional Papers, 6 December.
Mackley, B. and Heslop, T. (1979) The Aberdeen Formula: evaluation on the larger scale, Parts I, II and III. *Nursing Times*, Occasional Papers, 15 March, 22 March and 29 March.
Rhys Hearn, C. (1979) Comparison of Rhys Hearn method of determining nursing staff requirements with Aberdeen Formula. *International Journal of Nursing Studies*, **16,** 95-103.
Telford, W.A. (1979) *A method of determining nursing establishments*. East Birmingham Health District.

6

Measuring nursing workload and matching nursing resources

Monica Duncan, SRN, BSc(Hons), PG Cert Adult Ed, RNT, MBA, LIHSM, MBPS
Contracts Adviser, Royal Sussex County Hospital, Brighton

Defining nursing workload

To define nursing workload as the work which nurses do may seem to be a tautologous statement, but at least it is a start. Is it work where they can exercise professional discretion, or is it work shaped by tradition, custom and practice (White, 1985)? Nurses must be able to exercise professional discretion about their own workload, and be clear that nursing is a clinically based profession. There are many occasions when ward clerks and technology can take over clerical functions which in the past registered nurses have undertaken, as part of nursing activity.

Matching workload to resources

The way in which nurses choose to match themselves as a resource to the workload which they perceive to be a nursing workload depends both on individual values, attitudes and beliefs as well as management style, custom and practice. Shaping all of this is nurse education, which is changing radically, and valuable nursing resources would be wasted if nurses do not grasp the opportunities of the reformation of nurse education in the form of EN to RGN conversion courses and Project 2000 (UKCC, 1986; 1989). Despite the shortage of level 1 nurses, enormous obstacles are put in the way of level 2 registered nurses who wish to convert to level 1, and in many cases, legitimise the work they already undertake. This is hardly good resource management.

Measuring nursing workload and matching nursing resources

Why? Management tradition leads us to believe that nursing workload should be measured to assist with patient costing, provide management information and to assist in care planning and audit. Whilst these may be important reasons, purely on their own they infer 'scientific' management and are not the whole story.

Nurses must assess and predict, rather than measure retrospectively, nursing workload if they are to manage the resource of nurses as valuable employees. The demographic time bomb is ticking away, and an easy framework for considering its consequences is to remember that in 20 years time, there will be 20% fewer nurses and 20% more people aged 60 years and over (Beardshaw and Robinson, 1990). Nursing workload will increase, nursing resources will decrease and an inevitable consequence will be a sharp decline in the quality outcomes. Measuring nursing workload on an individual/client basis is important, and will be increasingly important in the future for three reasons:

1. Money will be following patients within the contractual framework, and money is used to buy nursing resources (DOH 1990).

2. Nurses will take an increasingly important role in the planning of care within Clinical Directorates, and assessing the consequences of evolving methods of treatment for their patients and clients. Resources must be planned as well as workload if a suitable quality of care is to be delivered.

3. Good quality care cannot be delivered if there are no nursing resources available to buy with the money. Nurses must be managed much more creatively than in the past. Nursing management must become really de-centralized, and not just nominally divisionalised within Clinical Directorates, so that they can respond more flexibly to both changing nursing practice and changing patterns of employment. Nursing workload has been measured in one form or another for quite a long time now, and much nursing management information has been gained. How much nursing management action has been returned? Events happen quickly in clinical areas and in the community, but the nurse who has responsibility for the delivery of nursing care rarely has the authority for deployment of nursing resources. If clinical responsibility is not firmly linked to real authority for resources, nurses will continue to leave the NHS (Beardshaw and Robinson, 1990).

Who?   Matching nursing workload to nursing resources would surely be accomplished more effectively if it were the same person doing it, or if at least it were done at the interface of nurses with their clients and patients. Historically, this has not been the case. It has usually been the ward sister, the community sister or in their absence their deputy measuring the nursing workload, with their line managers allocating resources. There is a gap, both in location and time about matching resources, and not surprisingly, the probability of matching the resources to the workloads decreases as this gap increases.

When?   Nursing workload is measured at the clinical level usually within 24 hours of delivering care, but planned resources are matched at best monthly, and at worst 3-yearly on establishment figures. Many ward sisters still do not know their staff allocation and vacancy factors and are unable to decide their own grade mix in terms of C, D, E and F grade nurses. Yet it is surely the ward sister who has the up-to-date knowledge about the nursing requirements of her patients and the capabilities of her staff.

Where? Nursing workload is measured in the clinical area and in clients' homes, and resources are matched in distant offices. Even then, the matching of resources tends to be in numbers of staff, grade mixes and whole time equivalents, with scant regard for the knowledge possessed by the individual nurses who will have to do the work. Few management units have a database of qualifications possessed by registered nurses on their staff. Not all nurse managers are up-to-date with the curricula of student nurses and the content of postregistration courses. Resources are not just about numbers and pairs of hands – knowledge is a resource which is often undervalued in nursing.

How? This is the most difficult part, and it is where grade mix must be addressed. Nursing workload is measured in terms of perceived demand for quality care, while nursing resources are measured in terms of quantity and skill mix of nurses available. The correlation between quantity and quality is not perfect, although it is an approximation. Broadly, there are two schools of thought on how to measure nursing workload and match resources.

The first method is the 'biological/managerial' perspective, which assumes that dependency arises primarily from the medical condition and physical dependence of patients or clients. The second method is the 'organisational' perspective, which assumes that organisational factors will alter dependency.

Biological/managerial perspective

One way of assessing patient demand is to categorize patients according to their requirements for nursing care. In many ways, this is entirely compatible with the nursing process, in that it asks what is to be done, how is it to be done and possibly by whom, although in the uni-professional model the 'whom' would relate solely to grade of nursing staff. This approach can be fraught with complexity, because not only are their differences in the statutory competencies of level 1 and level 2 registered nurses, but there are also sometimes conflicting job descriptions for these grades of nurses according to whether they are C, D, E or F Grade nurses (Nurses Pay Review Body, 1988).

A model of the main approaches to assessing nursing workload is shown in Figure 1.

Horizontal approach One approach could be termed a 'horizontal' approach from this model. A standard amount of nursing time by grade of nurse is determined, multiplied and weighted by the patient demand category to determine the staffing levels for the ward. Patient demand can be aggregated over time and this formula is the basis for traditional ward establishments. Time allocation, derived from nursing care plans,

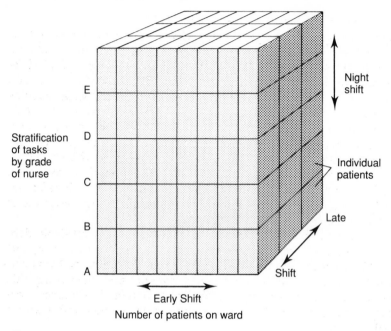

Figure 1. A model of approaches to assessing nursing workload.

forms the basis of many computerized nurse management systems, which then drive the rostering system to allocate and cost nursing time.

Vertical approach   A second approach could be termed a 'vertical' approach from this model. The nursing needs of each patient is assessed, assigning a level 1 registered nurse either to an individual patient or a small group of patients. It is less stratified than the 'horizontal' approach, but is nevertheless formula driven and forms the basis of many manual systems of calculating patient dependency such as GRASP, Monitor and Criteria For Care.

Professional judgement approach   A third approach is the 'professional judgement' method which also take a 'horizontal' approach. Patients are classified by level 1 registered nurses into agreed demand groups. The ward sister or nominated deputy is required to provide safe and acceptable care for all patients in their area. Professional judgement is used to negotiate variations from establishment to the number of nurses assigned to the ward, but establishment itself is derived from a formula. This approach forms the basis of such methods as the Telford Consultative Approach and the Brighton Method, which is no longer used. The crucial question when using the 'professional judgement' approach is whose professional judgement is considered important, the ward sister's or the Director of

Nursing Services' (Duberley and Norman, 1990)?

Using the biological/managerial perspective, an amount of nursing time is calculated and used to develop units of nursing time. Such units are based on how long it would take a given grade of nurse to undertake certain procedures with a patient or client. The procedures deemed necessary for the patient or client are based on physical needs, such as giving drugs, attending to hygiene and pre- or postoperative care. This is by no means a perfect solution, because there does not appear to be a purely linear relationship between the number of nursing staff and either the quantity or quality of nursing care received (Miller, 1984). However, it does follow that if insufficient nursing staff are available, then both the quality and quantity must be diminished. It is therefore an extremely useful tool to use to show what the likely outcomes are if insufficient nursing resources are available.

Units of nursing time are attractive in that they are quantifiable data which can be related to quality outcomes, are amenable to costing and can form the basis of 'what if' exercises for grade mix reviews. However, care must be taken to allow for indirect patient care when using this perspective. Units of nursing time according to patient dependency are a necessary but not sufficient factor to deliver both the required quantity and quality of nursing care.

Organisational theorists have been influential in linking job satisfaction to better performance. This link is shown in Figure 2.

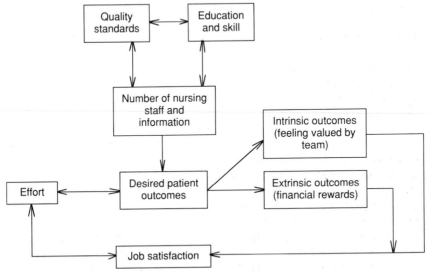

Figure 2. Inter-relationship of motivation and nursing resources.

Motivation appears to be the missing variable if the time aspect is used in isolation, and motivation takes account of the changes in the preparation of nursing students and their post registration development.

Post registration development is currently undergoing major changes in the light of the PREPP proposals. (UKCC, 1989). Team nursing and primary nursing are examples of nursing practice which may increase motivation within a more flexible structure. It is impossible to develop a universal definition of job satisfaction, but like nursing staff availability, if nursing job satisfaction is not there, again, both quality and quantity of nursing care are diminished. Useful proxy indicators of negative job satisfaction are staff turnover rates, sickness rates and absenteeism. These indicators also have a cost implication in terms of replacing staff.

Organisational perspective

The second method is the 'organisational' perspective. This method assumes that organisational factors will alter dependency, and so rather than illness and physical condition being the cause of dependency, they may be the result.

It is interesting to note that in nursing development units where organisational factors have been altered, there appears to be a marked improvement in patient or client dependency. Nurses in these areas have concentrated their efforts on the reduction of institutionalisation of their patients or clients, with impressive results despite often parsimonious budgets. The point about this method is that the nurses seem to have confidence in their clinical skills, and there is continuity of care, often based on primary nursing. Such continuity of care means that nurses can work with their patients or clients to establish goals, monitor whether these goals are achieved and alter the care accordingly.Implicit within this framework is an acknowledged relationship between the nurse and the patient or client, and flexibility on the part of the nurse.

Developing an appropriate method

There is no perfect universal solution, but there is a danger that if nurses fail to adopt a strategy themselves, someone will do it on their behalf. One possibility is a judicious mixture of the two approaches briefly outlined above, but probably not the adoption of either one in its pure form in all areas. The two approaches do at least offer some sort of continuum, and nurses could usefully apply their professional judgement to the clinical circumstances in which either one in its pure form would be appropriate, and when to mix them. They are not mutually exclusive and both have the considerable advantage of being undertaken by the nurse giving care to the patient. Gaps in time and location are overcome.

The quality of the environment must certainly be changed, such that nurses are able to use their valuable skills to the full. Automated rostering systems can enable ward sisters to work out their own 'best fit' to suit the individual requirements of the patients they are nursing, and have up-to-date information about the cost implications of their rotas. Ward sisters must have control of their own resources for which they need accurate, up-to-date knowledge about their own budgets. Nurse managers must develop strategic plans which link in with the overall organisation, and empower ward sisters with operational plans to manage resources according to their professional judgement. Measuring nursing workload and matching resources is essentially about closing the gap between plans and actions.

Knowledge is an important resource, and information technology can provide a fast framework to learn which nursing inventions have produced the best outcomes in given situations. Nursing knowledge can then be shared on an intra- and inter-disciplinary basis, so that we learn as individuals and collectively. There is a wealth of data about what nurses do with patients, and when, but it is sometimes difficult to turn that data into useable information about outcomes of nursing care. It is cumbersome and time consuming. Information technology can assist enormously in providing information to make informed decisions about measuring nursing workload and matching nursing resources. True professional judgement can only be acquired by learning, and learning may well mean changing both management and clinical practice. Matching nursing workload to nursing resources is achieved by planning and sharing information, and while some nurses may have to wait a little longer for the information technology which they so desperately need, all nurses can make a start on the cultural changes.

References

Beardshaw, V. and Robinson, R. (1990) New For Old: *Prospects For Nursing In The 1990s.* Kings Fund Institute, London.

DOH (1990) *Contracts For Health Services: Operational Principles.* DOH1, 4.

Duberley, J. and Norman, S. (1990) Nursing Data For Resource Management In: *Resource Management: The Leading Edge.* NHS Management Executive, London.

Gibbs, I., Mc Caughan, D. and Griffiths, M. (1991) Skill mix in nursing: A selective review of the literature. *Journal of Advanced Nursing,* **16**.

HMSO, (1984) *Working for Patients,* HMSO, London.

Miller, A. (1984) Nurse patient dependency: A review of different approaches with particular reference to elderly patients. *Journal Of Advanced Nursing,* **9**, 479–86.

Nurses Pay Review Body (1988) *For Nurses, Midwives, Health Visitors & Professions Allied To Medicine.* ELP 67, London.

UKCC (1989) *UKCC Post Registration Education and Practice Project.* United Kingdom Central Council for Nursing, Midwifery and Health Visiting, London.

UKCC (1986) *Project 2000: A New Preparation For Practice.* United Kingdom Central Council For Nursing, Midwifery and Health Visiting, London.

White, R. (1985) Political Regulators in British nursing political issues. In: *Nursing: Past, Present and Future,Vol 1.* John Wiley, London.

7

How to retain nurses

Hilary Shenton, RGN, Managing Director, Raine
Christine Hamm, RGN, Director, Raine

Staff recruitment and retention are major responsibilities for any manager, and require skills and organisation which may be new to many nurses. But, with their responsibilities as ward managers or community care managers, many ward sisters, charge nurses and community nurses are now involved in the appointment of new staff – and with the increasingly important issue of retaining them. Here we examine some of the issues surrounding staff retention, which will enable you to maintain good staffing levels, despite the increasing shortage of nurses.

Keeping staff

In an environment in which 30,000 nurses a year leave nursing altogether in Britain, and where the number of newcomers to nursing is falling along with the drop in the number of school-leavers, staff retention is a top priority. This is especially true in the particularly difficult specialties such as ITU and surgery, and in the cities. If the work environment is one in which nurses want to stay, obviously the need for recruitment will be minimised. It is also easier to attract staff to a stable working environment than to one in which everyone seems to be leaving.

Continuing education The provision of appropriate opportunities for continuing education for all staff is vital to enable existing employees to keep abreast of changes and developments, and to feel confident about their present professional role. It is also important to enable individuals to grow and develop their nursing skills, and for those who want to make career progressions to have the support and opportunity to do so. Employers who are seen to be offering appropriate continuing education, or providing the time for nurses to seek it outside, should have no difficulty in attracting staff – and keeping them. However, many employers pay only lip-service to the provision of continuing education, and many do not make the opportunities which *do* exist sufficiently well known to their staff.

The continuing education budget is often the first expenditure to be cut by cost-saving employers, but this is an expensive false economy. The introduction by the UKCC of a mandatory continuing education requirement for all nurses will help to sharpen the focus on this essential requirement for satisfactory employment.

Recognising and developing the skills of individuals All employees, at every level, need to feel that their skills are being recognised and, if possible, used. If they are not, the chances are that the individual will find another job where her skills and potential *are* recognised. Managers can only achieve this by *listening* to their staff and being open and supportive to their needs to develop. Regular appraisal meetings can be the most useful forum for this, but such meetings must be well conducted, and lead to feasible and appropriate action on the manager's part once the need is identified.

Flexible staffing arrangements In an inflexible environment, nurses will leave if their own time availability or home circumstances change in a way that cannot be accommodated by the employer. Often, only small changes may be needed to retain staff – the cost and inconvenience of which will be a lot less than the cost and inconvenience of trying to reappoint. The shortage of nurses is sharpening the focus of employers and employees on the need for more flexibility in patterns of employment. Job-sharing schemes and more creative provision for part-time work are being tried by some employers.

Accommodation and transport These are both big problems for nurses in the cities, particularly in London, where the cost of accommodation is so high. It is not unreasonable for a nurse in his or her late twenties to expect to start buying a flat and to furnish it, but this is almost impossible for most, unless they are willing to share. Travel and rent may cost as much as the outgoings on a mortgage, and many of the London hospitals are certainly losing staff for this reason. Nurses' homes must be of a sufficiently decent standard to be an attractive alternative, and even then may only be seen as a temporary arrangement by staff in their late twenties and beyond.

Some private hospitals are tackling this problem by buying houses some distance away and subsidising both the nurses' rent and travel. Many health authorities do have provision to offer interest-free loans for season tickets, and some have looked at subsidising car purchase. But such schemes must be made known to new and prospective staff. The pay review scales dictate the pay and regional weighting allowances which health authorities can offer nurses, but there is still scope for providing the extras – for example, taxis to and from the hospital for those on nights – which may make it possible for nurses to stay.

Security Most hospitals are publicly open places, and the level of petty crime is often a noticeable nuisance to all staff. Much more serious, though, is the apparently increasing risk of physical assault by patients, visitors and hospital intruders. If a hospital, community health centre or practice is based in an area known for such crimes, and if public transport is inefficient and relatively inaccessible, then the problem is compounded, particularly for staff coming off a late shift or going on night duty. A number of measures can be taken to ward off such crimes; several London hospitals have established 'help squads' which are on-call to deal with violent incidents within the hospital. One employer in London (not in health care) has issued all female staff with a loud and high-pitched personal alarm. Employers need to be aware of any such local problems and may need to be inventive with their approaches to the problem; they must be seen to really care about their staff.

Exit interviews

If the environment and conditions of employment reflect the genuine concern and care of an employer for staff, and if there is plenty of opportunity for staff to develop their professional skills and progress their careers, then the problems created by high staff turnover can be minimised. However, it is helpful to have some idea of the overall pattern of reasons staff have for leaving and this can be established by using 'exit interviews'. These must be undertaken by someone other than the individual's immediate manager – personnel staff would be more appropriate – and should briefly establish whether the real reasons for leaving are the same as those already given.

Over a period of months a pattern may emerge suggesting, for example, that a significant proportion of leavers felt that the shift structure was too rigid for their other commitments, or that there was 'no future' for them with their present employer. This is important information which must be acted on to reduce further unnecessary staff losses, and so improve the employer's chance of attracting newcomers.

Including the cost of staff time for interviews, secretarial and administrative time and advertising and possibly recruitment agency fees, it costs about £1,500 to recruit a staff nurse, and £2,000 to £3,000 to recruit a ward sister or charge nurse. These figures will be higher in the specialties where nurses are especially short in numbers. So it is clearly in the interests of a cost-conscious employer to reduce the level of recruitment required to maintain the agreed staffing levels.

8

Get the best from staff recruitment

Hilary Shenton, RGN, Managing Director, Raine

Christine Hamm, RGN, Director, Raine

However attractive the conditions of employment and working environment, and however good the morale, teamwork and opportunities for professional development at your place of work, people will inevitably leave and vacancies will need to be filled. With the current shortage of nurses, employers have to work hard to make their posts attractive. It is also important to make sure appointments are appropriate to the needs of existing staff. Here we will consider the issues arising from staff vacancies and how to fill them most efficiently.

Staff vacancy

Do you actually have a vacancy? If someone resigns, it is often the immediate reaction of their colleagues that the post must be refilled. But you do not necessarily have a vacancy when someone leaves: this can be an opportunity to restructure the department so that other staff have increased responsibilities which they are pleased to accept, or the post could be filled by promoting another member of staff, creating a vacancy, or an opportunity for restructuring, elsewhere. It is a good idea to spend at least a couple of days to consider the situation and to look at the needs and skills of others in the department and of the client group. It may be a good opportunity to offer another member of staff training so that they can develop the skills to fulfil the new post in a few months.

Seek out views The next step is critically important to the success of both the recruitment process and the future employment. The views and needs of *all* relevant colleagues, most importantly those who will be immediately responsible for the newcomer, *must* be sought. Their thoughts on the exact nature of the job, and the ideal skills, personal qualities and level of experience required are essential.

Increasingly, ward sisters and charge nurses are becoming actively involved in the recruitment process for their immediate ward staff. This involvement may make new demands, but will provide the ward managers themselves with the opportunity to build and maintain the team *they* feel is most appropriate for their clients and colleagues.

The staff to be involved in interviewing must also be identified and included in these discussions; there is no point in one group of interviewers shortlisting a candidate who is rejected by someone more senior with different views of the qualities required. Everyone's views must be known before the post is defined and advertised.

Internal or external appointment?

Again, the decision to consider all applicants, including existing staff, or to only look outside *must* be made before the post is advertised – and *everyone* in the relevant departments must be informed. If you decide to use this opportunity to bring in new skills from outside, it is demoralising for existing staff to apply and be rebuffed.

Similarly, if the post is open to internal applicants, they need to know, and should be given a deadline beyond which the post will be advertised externally, unless suitable candidates have applied.

Job descriptions should contain:
• Objectives of the job.
• Manager to whom the staff member will report.
• The individual duties of the job (list and detail no more than 12).
• Outline, for each of these duties, where responsibilities begins and ends.

Table 1. The job description

The ideal candidate:
• Level of experience required.
• Any special experience required.
• Personal qualities needed such as: flexibility of attitudes; leadership; problem-solving ability; ability to communicate well.
• Other requirements, such as flexibility to travel.

Table 2. The personnel specification

Job description and personnel specifications

Draw up a *brief* description of the job, based on the information and ideas pooled from relevant colleagues (Table 1) and also a list of qualities sought in the 'ideal' candidate (Table 2). These should be circulated to those involved with interviewing; the job description should also be sent to candidates called for interview. The interviewing team should also agree about the parts of both specifications on which they are willing to compromise: the absolutely ideal candidate rarely exists!

Advertising the vacancy

Advertising is not the only way of making a vacancy known, but it is the most effective way of reaching a wide selection of potential candidates.

Content   Put the minimum amount of information that will attract appropriate candidates to respond (Table 3). It is essential to describe the job clearly but briefly and to highlight particularly attractive opportunities or facilities (such as a professional development course which is available, or well-equipped ward). Include brief details of the *easiest possible* means of applying for the post. This is usually a (correct!) telephone number, and the name of someone friendly and helpful who will be at the extension given (check that they are not on holiday or on a course during the week after the advertisement is placed) and can get an application in the post first class to enquirers the same day.

Put the minimum information to attract response:
- Job title.
- A sentence to stimulate interest and make potential candidates want the job.
- Details of the easiest means of applying.
- Salary grade.
- Closing date.

Table 3. The advertisement

Design   In magazines where there are many advertisements, a large advertisement will attract more attention, and the inclusion of a border or logo may also help to catch the eyes of potential applicants. Advertising is expensive, but so is bridging the gap between staff. Disruption and increased workload on existing staff should also be considered.

Timing   How urgent is the re-appointment? If the time scale is not at panic proportions, it is probably advisable to avoid advertising just before bank holiday weekend. If another post is coming up you may decide to delay advertising for a week or two so the two can be advertised together in a bigger space. On the other hand, you may feel it would boost the morale of existing staff to advertise early.

Choose the right medium   The only valid measure to assess the effectiveness of magazines or newspapers is the response rate to the advertisements you place. It is also important that the applicants who respond are appropriate for the post, but your wording for the advertisement should ensure this. If you want and need good responses *do not* place your advertisement in a publication where you know you get a very low response rate. You may decide, however, that you want to be seen to be supporting a particular group, and place the advertisement in its journal. Local papers can also be useful.

Handling the applications

If possible, let every applicant know that their application has arrived and is being considered. Inform anyone whose application is obviously inappropriate *straight away,* so that they can get on with more appropriate applications. Once the closing date has passed, let your interviewing team draw up a shortlist for interview. Invite interviewees as early as possible for interview and an informal visit; if candidates have a long distance to travel, these could both be on the same day.

Informal visits   These *must* be informal, and not used as an extra interview. They should give the candidate the opportunity to assess the working environment and the job in a relaxed atmosphere. Their questions should be answered by someone who is enthusiastic about the work; preferably *not* by the person who is leaving.

Interviews   Decide who will be interviewing and how long the interviews will be and inform the candidates of this at the start. The interviewing panel should be kept as small as possible – preferably no more than three people – and interviewers must have the views and requirements and the trust of their relevant colleagues.

It is not easy to assess all the professional skills and personal qualities of a candidate in an interview, but it is possible to get a clear idea of the individual's appropriateness for the job, assessed against the qualities you have identified for the 'ideal' candidate. You need to assess their professional skills and level of motivation, which can be done by asking them to talk about their last (or present) job. Ask what they enjoyed most and least, and what they could handle, given more training. Ask them to identify their training needs, as this will help to build a picture of what they would like most to be doing.

Assessing personal qualities such as leadership and problem-solving ability is difficult, but asking how they have handled problems in previous posts will help. Referees' reports are also important here.

Do not be afraid of 'digging too deep' in an interview: as long as you do not ask unfair personal questions, it is reasonable to find out about the candidate in some depth. After all, it is important for them that they find themselves in the 'right' job, too.

References
At least two references should be sought, one from the current or last employer, and one from a previous employer (or, if newly qualified, from the candidate's school of nursing). An *employer's* reference (even from a non-nursing employer if the candidate was not previously in nursing) is more valuable than that from a colleague (Table 4).

Ask referees for:
- Statement of the candidate's duties.
- Length of employment.
- Sickness and absenteeism record.
- Reliability.
- Ability as a team member.
- Professional conduct.
- Other qualities and skills.

Table 4. The reference

It is often possible to gain more frank analysis and information and depth from a referee by telephoning them. Most people are now willing to give references in this way; give them the option to think about it and telephone you back. You could ask for a written reference, and then telephone the referee for a more detailed discussion. Always check that the candidate is happy for you to contact their referees before doing so, and work fast.

Offering the job

Once the interviewers have agreed upon the candidate for the post, act fast and offer the post, subject to satisfactory references. This could be done on the same day as the interview, and, if they have already had an informal visit, you should expect an immediate (or reasonably quick) response. Do not wait until the references are in – you may lose the candidate to another employer.

Making the appointment

Once the candidate accepts the job, keep up the momentum and get the starting date agreed, uniform measured and holidays booked. Write immediately to confirm the appointment, terms, conditions and starting date; people are reluctant to hand in their notice until they have the job offer in writing. Also, inform the other applicants as quickly as possible.

It is hoped that if these suggestions for recruitment are followed and some of the ideas for retaining staff acted upon, it should be possible to build and maintain reasonable staffing levels – even in the specialties where nurses are few and far between, and in work places located in the heart of cities.

9

Job sharing can take the strain out of recruitment

Ann Shuttleworth, BA
Editor, Professional Nurse

Shortage of labour costs huge sums of money in industry – in health care it costs lives. The projected shortage of nurses is already biting in some specialties and areas, and it is essential for health authorities to retain the staff they have, and attract more recruits – and as the number of 18-year-olds drops, different kinds of recruits. However, unlike industry, they cannot simply pay higher salaries to attract people, so they have to find new ways to persuade people to nurse – ways that compete with the money industry has to offer.

Health authorities have begun to move towards greater flexibility in working hours, to try to attract those people – mainly women – whose other commitments make them unable to undertake full-time work. Part-time work is often characterised by low pay, job insecurity, poor promotion prospects and the lack of fringe benefits. Far more appealing to many is job sharing, an idea which began in the early 1970s as more women decided they wanted families without giving up their careers. They often found the part-time work available was low paid and low skilled, and at a lower level than they had been used to.

A voluntary arrangement

Job sharing is an arrangement whereby two (or more) people voluntarily share one full-time post, sharing salary and benefits between them according to the hours they work. As long as each one works 16 or more hours a week, they are eligible for employment protection. Within this definition, job sharing is completely flexible in how the job is shared, and is at the convenience of the employees and employers concerned. Most people suggest a job share with a partner already in mind, although some have been put in touch with each other after applying for jobs advertised as suitable for a job share. Normal contracts are usually suitable with appropriate amendments, but sharers may wish to add clauses to cover such eventualities as one wishing to leave.

Advantages

There are many advantages in job sharing, both for employees and employers. The most obvious advantage for the employee is the opportunity to work part-time while retaining the advantages and security of a full-time post. This alone makes job sharing attractive both to nurses wishing to work part-time without moving to a lower grade and those who have taken a career break and want part-time work at the grade they had previously attained.

Job sharing also gives more opportunities for jobs to reflect individuals' interests and skills than part-time work. The increased free time is not only a chance to care for children – it can also be used for the pursuit of research or study interests. In a profession as potentially stressful and demanding as nursing, the opportunity to work in a responsible position only part-time alleviates these problems, while job sharers can offer mutual support and different expertise.

There are also numerous advantages for employers (Buchan, 1987). Trained staff can be retained and are less likely to suffer from job related stress, a major cause of absenteeism. Voluntary job-sharers are also likely to have a high level of commitment since they have shown a positive desire for their job by arranging the job-share, rather than opting for a more easily attained post. They are also likely to be more flexible and able to provide additional cover in peak periods. Working shorter hours, they have often been found to be more productive and able to sustain higher levels of activity.

Disadvantages

While the advantages to both employees and employers make job-sharing attractive, it does have potential disadvantages. Employees' earnings will obviously be limited and promotion prospects may be decreased. A tendency has also been found in job sharers to work more than their half-time, and they may experience some loss of job satisfaction. They will certainly have to ensure their managers do not try to give them too much work and the post is subject to the usual appraisal systems. Sharing the control and responsibilities of the job may cause problems, and must usually be resolved by compromise.

Employers have cited potential disadvantages from their point of view, but in practice these are not always significant (Buchan, 1987). The cost of employing two people – providing uniforms and training, and paying for time spent together in handover is higher, but National Insurance may actually be lower if the post attracts a gross pay of less than £350 a week. The handover time is likely to be minimal, and it has been argued that it leads to increased planning and efficiency.

Job sharers' managers may have to spend more time in supervision and work allocation, although no recorded schemes have reported this as a problem. Staff supervised by the job sharers may find difficulty being accountable to two people, especially if they have different ideas on organisation. Problems may also occur if one sharer wishes to leave.

These disadvantages can be overcome given commitment from those involved, as Judith Lathlean (1987) found in evaluating a job shared ward sister post at the Charing Cross Hospital in London. The sisters found initial resistance from their staff, who knew one of the sisters well and the other not at all. Hackney Job Share, an external organisation, came in to explain to the staff about job sharing and diffuse some of their negative feelings. The first few months involved the sisters in high levels of communication in setting up systems, and they found they had to compromise to reach workable agreements on issues in which they differed. Once systems were operating, the ward settled down and the staff gradually became more supportive and understanding.

While the job share described by Lathlean was not without difficulties, on the whole it was successful and illustrates that job sharing is possible for jobs with managerial responsibilities. Lathlean recommends that health authorities consider job sharers in more posts, and take the initiative in creating opportunities for employees to job share.

New ways to Work (NWTW) is an organisation committed to advising people on job sharing and other flexible working ideas, such as annual hours and taking career breaks. Started in 1979 as a voluntary organisation, NWTW are now funded by the London Boroughs Grant Scheme to advise both employees and employers. They are currently involved with the Royal Institute of Public Administration in designing a course on job sharing aimed specifically at health authorities.

Health authority interest

They say health authorities are starting to take a little more interest in job sharing, but they are still lagging behind local authorities in actively promoting job sharing schemes. NWTW feel that health authorities are finding it something of a hurdle to start encouraging job sharers, and most of those employed by health authorities say they have had difficulty in negotiating their posts. There are exceptions, however, including one manager who advertised a post specifically as a job share, and another who has several health visitor job share partnerships.

Obviously, some posts will adapt more easily to a job share than others, and will be more easily broken down. NWTW say, however, that most jobs can be successfully shared, given commitment and flexibility from all concerned. Difficult managerial posts have been shared successfully, allowing people with years of experience to continue to work at the level they are qualified for, rather than leaving employment altogether or working in lower grade jobs. They say it is essential for professional organisations to get involved in encouraging job sharing, as people are most likely to contact them for advice.

Job sharing may not answer all the problems of nurse recruitment, but it could certainly tap an unused and probably frustrated pool of experienced ex-nurses unwilling to return to part-time work at a lower level than they left, and retain many who wish to devote some time to other commitments. If it is to live up to its full potential, health authorities and the nursing unions will have to become more active in publicising the idea and helping potential sharers negotiate their posts.

References
Buchan (1987) A shared future. *Nursing Times,* **83,** 4.
Lathlean, J. (1987) *Job sharing a ward sisters post.* Riverside Health Authority, London.

Useful addresses
New Ways to Work
309 Upper Street
London N1 2TY
Tel: 071-226 4026.

Hackney Job Share Project
380 Old Street
London
Tel: 071-739 0741.

10

Part-time staff: a blessing in disguise?

Jean Fisher, SRN, ONC
Clinical Teacher, St Michael's Hospice, Bartestree, Hereford

As a ward sister with a full-time staff of four, including myself, out of a full complement of 12, to cover the 'day-time' hours from 07.30 to 21.30 hours, all the pleasures and pains of managing part-time staff can certainly be said to be mine. In this particular setting of a small, purpose-built hospice, which is totally charity-run, the stresses and strains – as well as the job satisfaction – encompass both the high and low of nursing morale.

The particular stress encountered here is in coping with pain, and fear, anger and desperation in patients, and also in dealing almost daily with bereaved families. To counteract that the staff has the satisfaction of usually being able to help relieve suffering with good symptom control and that most precious gift – time. More often than not, the nurse may only need an extra five minutes with patients to really make them comfortable or to find out what they are really frightened of.

Those few extra minutes are often just not available to nurses, but to the patient may mean the difference between good nursing and the extra special 'caring' that hospices are all about. All nurses – whether they work in a hospital or hospice – want to give those minutes and they become frustrated when they see less and less time available to spend with patients due to constant pressure and staff shortages. Using part-time staff may provide part of the solution for several problems, including this one.

Increased flexibility
For the employer, one of the greatest advantages of using part-time staff must be increased flexibility. At the hospice all nursing staff (except those employed on the nursing bank) work full shifts in an effort to increase continuity and teamwork. However, there is no doubt that even more flexibility can be obtained (and some considerable financial saving made) by staff working part shifts at peak hours, ie, mornings and 'twilight' shifts. My view is that staff commitment and participation is higher when they are at work for a whole shift and can take part in ward reports, case conferences and decision making.

Almost all continuing education in the form of lectures, video viewing and so on take place in the afternoon during the overlap period. Very few staff off duty at 13.00 hours would be able, or willing, to return at 14.30 hours for a lecture or ward staff meeting. The other important factor in the use of full shift patterns is that staff can be given back 'time owing' during the overlap period. It is known that nurses often work extra time. It is also well known that, more often than not, they do so willingly, to maintain the level of nursing care given to their patients. It is not usually possible for them to be paid for this time. However, this commitment should not be taken for granted – commitment is a two-way process, and therefore 'time off in lieu' should be given at mutual convenience to the unit and the member of staff. The pressure in many areas today usually prevents this, and the extra frustration upon so many others could well become the straw that breaks the camel's back. But 'time off in lieu' might even encourage staff to come in on a day off sometimes for a lecture if that time could be given back during a quiet period.

The other flexibility of part-time staff is that, if necessary, one can *occasionally* ask a part-time nurse to cover an extra part-time shift when unforeseen staffing problems occur. This would obviate the need for agency staff, who are expensive and provide less continuity of care. It is important that staff who are willing to do extra time do not feel that they *have* to do so and that they are not taken advantage of by being asked on a regular basis.

Stress
Stress levels in part-time staff are undeniably lower, which in the hospice situation is vital. The extra time for 'real life' means nurses are more refreshed and have more to offer when they are at work. But what about the effect the number of part-time staff has on the stress levels of their full-time colleagues? In fact, it may *increase* their stress levels a little, in that the onus to provide continuity lies more heavily upon them. However, in many ways this can only be another recommendation for good documentation and the implementation of the nursing process with full-time staff coordinating the nursing teams.

The added stress of working part-time is that it can become more difficult to make useful relationships with patients and their families. However, this may be an advantage if it makes staff less complacent about making contact with patients and relatives. Clinical observations may be much more acute from part-time staff as they have more time away from work and therefore see changes in situations more clearly than staff who are there five days a week.

The small details of the smooth running of the ward are those that break down at times. When the part-time staff nurse hardly ever works the third Tuesday in the month and is therefore not usually required to order stores . . . except when sister is on a day off and the full-time staff nurse is sick . . . then problems can arise. Like most problems there is usually a solution.

Another advantage for employers in taking on part-time staff is ease of recruitment. Present staff shortages and recruitment problems highlight the outdated historical ideal of nurses being single women, working full-time on a vocational basis, with no life away from work. It is now becoming apparent that few nurses fit into this category today. There are many nurses leaving the profession, or not returning after a break, because of management failure to make it either feasible or acceptable to do so. Hopefully, the increase in crêche facilities, 'back to nursing' courses and the moves towards improved continuing education in nursing (UKCC, 1990), together with flexibility of employer and employee will put this situation to rights. If the idea of job sharing (Cole, 1987) does spread, many high calibre senior nurses may be able to stay in or return to their profession.

Common sense

Most of the staff at St Michael's Hospice are married, and some have children. As their sister, I am always grateful for their common sense approach and skills of empathy as, being younger and single, I still have much to learn in certain situations. If nurses seriously want to take the abnormality and mystique out of ward situations (in hospital, nursing home or wherever the wards may be) they should aim to make them as much like the outside world as possible. This means a good staff mix (single and married as well as more men). The single staff also have their own skills. They may often have new ideas and practices to share, which may be varied as single nurses tend to be less settled. Often, married staff – unless their partners are in the Services – stay in one area for a much longer span of time. Herein lies the answers to a manager's prayer – married staff can provide ongoing continuity and single staff bring new ideas. They can bring the best (or perhaps prevent the worst) from Oxford, East Grinstead or Outer Mongolia!

Skill mix is not just a question of the ratio of trained to untrained staff but also of age group, background and professional expectations. A unit where the turnover of staff is as high as that of the patients is as difficult to manage as one where no one has moved for years. All ward sisters know at some time the frustration of training a bright young staff nurse only to find that once you make progress and she becomes able to be your right hand, the obligatory six months or one year is up and she is off to the next rung of the ladder. We have all done it ourselves and accept its inevitability, but there is no doubt that a nucleus of staff who have been in the team for a while makes for smooth running. The management skills required then are to maintain commitment and prevent staleness and the old adage, 'We always do it this way'. Also, it prevents exclusivity and a clique formation that precludes newcomers from being accepted as part of the team. A clear and agreed ward philosophy should help to prevent these occurring, but the situation needs constant and careful monitoring (Teasdale, 1987; DHSS, 1986; Mallin, 1987; Moores, 1986).

Commitment

Diminished level of commitment among part-time staff is an often quoted problem but is, I suspect, a fallacious one. Certainly among my own staff, the level of caring and commitment is as high in part-time as in full-time staff. The personal areas of responsibility and accountability have never been more clearly stated within the nursing profession and this can only decrease the degree of complacency which exists in some members of various professions. The days of the ward sister 'carrying the can' for every occurrence is being replaced at last. This alone must increase the level of motivation in most trained staff. It may be more difficult for part-time staff, particularly those working on night duty, to participate in continuing education, as often the reason for doing night duty is to dovetail family commitments and work. My own staff seem to have most amenable partners, mothers, neighbours, cousins and aunts who can take care of children for a day to allow them to attend a study day or conference.

Motivation in giving care to an agreed standard is not, or should not be, a problem. Most nurses have high personal standards for bedside care. Why are so many leaving the NHS at the moment? Not because their own standards are inadequate, (or at least only in a very small number of cases) but because they feel they cannot practise at what they consider an acceptable standard. It is the frustration, stress and constant pressure which is driving so many out into the private sector, or abroad, or, most sadly of all, out of nursing altogether. Most nurses want to do their best for patients whether they are on duty for two days a week or five. Certainly the bank staff employed by the hospice, who may come in for a half shift to cover sickness perhaps only once a month, give excellent care to patients and their families (West Dorset H.A., 1987).

I am sure that the level of commitment among staff is high when they are in a position to give good care, as part of a caring team, supported by all tiers of whichever structure they are working within. Staff whose input of care is being respected and appreciated will have higher morale. They will give of their best, perhaps not in every shift – which none of us can – but in a more than acceptable majority.

A valuable part to play

Part-time staff have a valuable part to play in any nursing team. They can provide continuity, stability, maturity and empathy, and enhance the 'normality' of ward environment sought by many team leaders.

The situation in which I work may be said by some to be ideal. It is a small unit, with a small team which works very closely together. It is not attached to a hospital and is not bound by the conservative and short-term views found in some health authorities. The system of part-time staff working full-shift days has been most successful. Working in partnership with patients (Teasdale, 1987) has to begin with partnership with colleagues and managers. Accepting the holistic approach to patient care may well have to begin by accepting a holistic approach to staff needs. Then perhaps better staff will be recruited and retained for longer and they will give better patient care.

References
Cole, A. (1987) Job sharing – partners in time. *Nursing Times, 83,* 40.
DHSS (1986) *Mix and match: a review of nursing skill mix.* DHSS, London.
Mallin, H. and Wright-Warren, P. (1987). Review mix and match. *Senior Nurse,* **6, 3.**
Moores, B. (1986) Review mix and match document. *Journal of Advanced Nursing,* **12,** 6.
Teasdale, K. (1987) Partnership with patients. *The Professional Nurse,* **2,** 40, 397-9.
UKCC (1990). *The PREPP Report.* UKCC, London.
West Dorset H.A. (1987) *Standards of Care Quality.* West Dorset Health Authority.

11

Can continuing education ease the nursing shortage?

Janet D. Duberley, MSc, SRN, RSCN, RCNT, Dip. Adv. Nurs. Stud.
Regional Nurse, Education and Practice, South West Thames Regional Health Authority

Nursing is facing major problems as the shortage of nurses begins to bite, and since there is no single reason for the shortage, there can be no single solution. It seems, however, that continuing professional education (CPE) is currently being used as the panacea to cure all the ills of staff recruitment and retention. I would suggest that at best it could serve as 'First Aid', at worst it could exacerbate the problem unless structural and organisational changes are also made.

What is continuing education?

Generally considered to be a 'good thing' CPE has an aura of common knowledge. However, common knowledge, like common sense, is remarkably uncommon, so I would like to explore the concept of CPE.

Houle (1980) says it relates to a dynamic concept of professionalisation with the ultimate aim "to convey a complex attitude made up of a readiness to use the best ideas and techniques of the moment, but also to expect that they will be modified or replaced. Everyone must expect constant change and with it new goals to be achieved and new understanding and skill to be mastered". This preparation for change is rather nebulous, so what does it mean in real terms? The American Nurses Association (ANA) defines CPE as "learning activities intended to build upon the educational and experimental basis of the professional nurse for the advancement of practice, education, administration, research or theory development to the end of improving the health of the public."

This definition contains a sense of what Houle calls the dynamic concept of professionalisation – the major focus builds on what has gone before to improve the public's health. However, what the learning activities might be is open to interpretation – the definition focuses on the different activities of nursing practice, education, administration and research. There is no mention of the *what* or *how* the public's health might be improved. In comparison, the American Medical Association (AMA, 1979) says "continuing medical education is composed of any education and training which serves to maintain, develop or increase the knowledge, interpretive and reasoning proficiencies, appropriate technical skills, professional performance standards or ability for interpersonal relationships that a physician uses to provide the service needed by patients or the public.''

This comprehensive and thought provoking definition does not relate solely to 'keeping up-to-date', nor does it focus on how medicine is practised, but to maintaining, developing and increasing intellectual and cognitive skills as well as psychosocial and psychomotor skills. The definition's goals relate to the ideals of professionalism – the possession of a unique body of knowledge – but also, and especially, to the expert application of that knowledge through the development of the intellectual skills of interpretation and reasoning.

How do employers see CPE?

How do these definitions compare with the way employers might view CPE? The type of CPE supported and promoted by employing organisations give us a clear idea of their perspective. In 1985 Rogers conducted a national review of CPE in nursing, and found a tremendous amount fell primarily into three categories:

- In-service training. Staff orientation/introduction, policy dissemination.
- Clinical updating. Issues and trends in clinical practice and practical skills training.
- Post registration clinical role preparation. Six to 12 month courses in clinical nursing.

The activities most heavily supported and prevalent in all organisations were in-service training. These were well planned, with records of attendance kept in many cases, especially for those on fire and safety policies. Clinical updating activities were also present in most organisations, but tended to be less well planned and coordinated. Post registration clinical role preparation was provided where appropriate experience was available, but not all experience supported clinical courses.

These findings suggest that employees value the activities they see as contributing to the achievement of their organisational goals – providing a high quality, effective service. To fulfill these goals, staff must be aware of the environment, geography, personnel, operational and safety policies. Surely nurses' clinical knowledge and skills should have at least equal standing?

How do practitioners see CPE?

From the practitioner's point of view, the meaning of CPE may be determined by her or his age, previous experience of preregistration and continuing education and career goals. Cervero (1981) identified four major factors motivating doctors to participate in CPE:

- To maintain and improve professional competence and service to patients.

- To understand oneself as a professional.
- To interact with colleagues.
- To enhance personal and professional position.

The practitioner's view of CPE is different to those of the profession and the employers. It retains the service ideal but focuses more on the individual – CPE has a personal meaning as well as a professional one.

Potential areas of conflict

It is generally believed that responsibility for the continuing high quality of professional practice is equally shared by the profession, the employer and the practitioner, but their priorities may differ. The profession wants to advance its position in service to the public, and the employer wants to provide a high quality and cost-effective service to the public. The practitioner is pulled four ways – serving the public; fulfilling professional ideals; serving the employer, and meeting (or not meeting) personal goals.

This fourth component can cause real conflict. In undertaking CPE and acquiring more knowledge and skills, the practitioner may come to expect more of professional practice and of its financial remuneration. However, while enhancement of the individual's position featured in practitioners' goals, it did not feature in those of the profession or the employer, so the practitioner may not have a forum in which to practise these newly acquired skills or to be recompensed for them.

This conflict, I would suggest, is reflected in current nurse staffing problems. Nurses are expressing frustration, they have a poor self-image, and this contributes to high staff turnover and wastage. Obviously, pay levels and the high cost of living in the south of England have an effect, but I believe that even if the problems over pay were to be rectified tomorrow, the frustration would be evident again in a very short time. Why? Because pay is not the whole problem.

Over the last three years, the nursing shortage has assumed considerable political significance. People are anxious to know why nurses are leaving the profession. Analysis of the 1981 census data in two regional health authorities demonstrates that only 20 per cent of people holding nursing qualifications are currently employed in the profession. This suggests there is not a shortage of nurses, but a shortage of nurses employed in the profession. This in turn suggests there is something about the workplace or practice of nursing that makes people leave.

In 1986, Oxford District Health Authority, concerned about high staff turnover among clinical nurses conducted an extensive study to find the cause of nurses' dissatisfaction. The overwhelming response was that nurses felt unable to provide the care they believed their patients deserved. This was partly due to low staffing levels, but also due to frustration. Having trained in the profession, nurses were increasingly less able to practise nursing – their time was spent doing other things.

Waite (1986) undertook a national survey for the RCN, which came up with similar findings. Nurses who had left the health service or who had seriously considered doing so reported not feeling they were doing a worthwhile job; being unable to use their initiative; poor promotion prospects; not being valued. These sentiments indicate a restricted framework which does not allow nurses to practise nursing. Their expertise is not valued either in monetary terms or in years of professional practice, and they do not have a structure in which they can function as expert practitioners.

When nurses feel frustrated in their profession, they have a number of options. Many simply continue in their frustration – they have a poor image of both themselves and their profession, and take no action 'because it wouldn't make any difference'. Others use their frustration as an impetus for change. These nurses may seek greater challenge by changing jobs within clinical nursing, thus contributing to the high staff turnover in the profession. Others may pursue further education.

Since Rogers' survey of CPE opportunities in 1985, and the recognition of the nursing shortage there has been a great deal of investment in CPE. In some cases it has been used as a carrot to attract and retain nurses, but unfortunately it often only works for the duration of the course. On completion of the course, many nurses either change jobs or leave the profession altogether. I believe this is because employing authorities do not consider how to use the newly acquired skills, which means the nurses remain in their state of frustration and have no alternative but to consider a job change. While by no means all job changes within nursing can be attributed to this, the reality is that with few exceptions, employers have no structure for recognition or acceptance of clinical nurses who pursue education for advanced clinical practice.

Could a structure be created?

In the USA, clinical career structures have developed in a different way than in this country. Using a theoretical model of skill acquisition, Benner (1984) identified distinguishable differences in the competence of nurses with different levels of expertise. This has provided a rationale for the development of a career ladder within clinical nursing. Benner describes five stages of clinical development: novice; advanced beginner; competent; proficient and expert. The latter three are relevant here.

The competent practitioner   This practitioner is typified by the nurse who has been doing the same or a similar job for two or three years. She demonstrates a mastery of and ability to cope with the many contingencies of clinical nursing. Nursing care is conscious, deliberately planned and effective.

The proficient practitioner   This practitioner perceives situations as wholes rather than as aspects of the whole. Previous experience enables the proficient practitioner to recognise when the expected normal picture does not materialise. Decision making is improved because the nurse has a perspective on which of the many aspects are the important ones. Proficient performance is usually found in nurses who have worked in similar clinical settings for three to five years.

The expert practitioner   This practitioner has an intuitive grasp of clinical situations. Her enormous background of experience enables her to home in on the accurate region of the problem without time consuming consideration of a wide range of alternative problems and solutions. While the expert practitioner appears not to rely on analytical principles, highly skilled analytical ability is necessary for those situations in which the nurse has no previous experience.

Implications for staff development

In describing levels of clinical expertise, Benner has provided the basis for a clinical career structure based on clinical competence, rather than managerial criteria as we have at present. But such defined career rungs have implications for staff development and continuing education in general. We must re-examine the goals and practice of CPE. It is the possession of cognitive, intellectual and interpretive skills that distinguishes the expert from the competent practitioner. CPE must address how it will facilitate the development of these skills.

However, as stated earlier, education and the acquisition of skills may not assist the retention of qualified nurses. These skills must be valued and recognised by employers. The current review of nursing manpower in terms of demand, supply and skill mix must take on a broader meaning than simply qualified:unqualified ratios. An examination of the level of skill requirements in clinical areas lends itself to the concept of clinical career ladders, to the proper use of scarce nursing resources and to proper levels of remuneration for clinical expertise. Unless this happens, CPE will only serve as First Aid. CPE should support the development of professional practice, but in association with the aims and goals of employing authorities.

References

AMA (1979) Proceedings of the 128th Annual Convention of the Council of Medical Education. July 22-26. Council on Medical Education, Report C.

Benner, R. (1984) *From Novice to Expert*. Addison Wesley, Mento Park, California.

Cervero, R. (1981) A factor analytical study of physicians' reasons for participating in continuing education. *Medical Education*, **56**, July, 29-34.

Houle, C.O. (1980) *Continuing Learning in the Professions*. Jossey-Bess, San Francisco.

Oxford District Health Authority (1986) DHA Member Report (Unpublished).

Rogers, J. (1987) *Continuing Professional Education for Qualified Nurses*. Austen Cornish Publishers and Ashdale Press, London. (Research carried out in 1985.)

Waite, R. and Hutt, R. (1987) *Attitudes, Jobs and Mobility of Qualified Nurses*. A report for the RCN. Institute of Manpower Studies, Brighton.

12

Building confidence: a development programme for newly qualified staff nurses

Sue Thame, BA
Independent Management Trainer, Pinner, Middlesex

When you first qualified as a staff nurse, would you have welcomed yet more training? The findings of a review conducted by Hillingdon Health Authority (1986) clearly showed that one of the major causes of dissatisfaction among nurses was the lack of training and education immediately after qualification. The authority therefore made it a priority to pioneer a development programme for newly qualified staff nurses.

Setting up the programme

In June 1987 Barbara Baker, an experienced nursing tutor, was appointed Senior Nurse Professional Development, with a remit to create a programme for newly qualified staff nurses. The key purpose was to prepare a more confident and skilled staff nurse for the future, and help with retention and recruitment.

The programme outline suggested a two year course (later amended to 14 months) and newly qualified staff nurses would be recruited both internally and nationally. They would be offered an attractive package: five days off-the-job training in management and interpersonal skills; three-monthly study days in their own selected subject areas; on-the-job support and counselling from a full-time nursing tutor; on-going written assignments; and planned four-monthly rotations between different wards. The nurses' individual development would be based on their own assessments of their areas of greatest need, drawn from a broad spectrum of learning objectives. Their choices would·be made in consultation with the nurse tutor and their nurse managers. The heart of the programme was to be the on-the-job counselling and support. This programme outline has been fully implemented.

My involvement in this project came about by invitation from Barbara Baker. I was already working with Hillingdon on an extended programme for nurses to improve their communication skills. Mounting such a major project within tight deadlines could have been more than just a headache – it could have spelt disaster. The coordination and communication required was extensive – not least finding, within a year,

30 nurse managers who would enthusiastically accept and train a revolving nursing staff. The Authority, however, organised itself efficiently by establishing a steering group that could be effective across the district, co-opting people who were enthusiastic, believed in the basic concept and could communicate across the hospital complex. The steering group had to influence people with hard facts and persuasive argument to obtain the resources and commitments required.

Since the new programme was to be based on findings of Rogers and Lawrence (1987) it was essential that all those involved agreed the basic rationale behind it. There were also all the politics of organisational life that must be attended to, in order to manage an innovation like this successfully. Too often, the power games for managing innovation are dealt with *sotto voce*, as if it is not quite 'naice' to speak and think the politics of a situation through clearly. The steering group's composition ensured the delicacies of diplomacy would be addressed. Each hospital and the community was represented on the group by a senior nursing manager. There was a senior representative from the nurse planning committee, a tutor from post basic education and Barbara Baker herself.

The first programme

The first programme began in February 1988 and we have some measure of the impact on the initial five participants, all of whom have found the programme a positive experience. Perhaps the most noticeable strength of the programme is its clear learning objectives. For the first time there is a full picture of what kinds of development a newly qualified staff nurse requires, with real support in attaining those aims.

At the start of the course the nurses are given a 20 page document on guidelines and objectives of the course (Baker, 1987). Daunting? Perhaps – until they see and understand the treasures it offers. It is their route to learner-centred development, and to taking charge of their own development. There is a comprehensive description of the aims and structure of the course and a full listing of the range of learning objectives they can choose to pursue for themselves (Table 1). Later they receive a profiling instrument to help them assess their starting point across all the learning objectives – to select their priorities for development. The evaluation forms, which enable the nurses to monitor their own progress, are used at the end of their ward allocations.

This comprehensive documentation ensouls the philosophy being pioneered at Hillingdon, and if my reading of the literature is correct, they are pioneers within the NHS as a whole too. At the core of their approach is the belief, from their own experience, that an effective hospital service must be based on a workforce constantly aware of the need to learn and change. Responsibility of this kind must be shared between employer and employee, because neither, alone, can know what is best. Both sides must interact to identify individual and group learning needs and to meet those needs. Nurses have traditionally been spoon-fed their basic

---

Six Key Aims

1. Interpersonal skills
At the end of the course the nurse will have an appreciation of the factors involved in good communications and an increased awareness of self and others.
Four specific objectives are listed
eg, use a problem solving approach
: thinking skills
: transactional analysis

2. Management of patient care
At the end of the course the nurse will understand the principles of clinical management and the role and responsibility of the staff nurse.
The nurse will be able to draw up and administer the individual nursing care plans based on the nursing process following the pattern of assessing needs, planning nursing care programmes, delivery of the care and evaluation.
Seven specific objectives are listed
eg, identify features of stress and anxiety in patients and relatives
: signs of stress
: symptoms of stress
: stress in hospitals

3. Teaching and assessing
The nurses will have an understanding of the learning process and a basic knowledge and skill in teaching and assessing.
Fourteen specific objectives are listed
eg, identify the factors which stimulate and sustain motivation in learners
: needs, drives, motives
: need to achieve and
fear of failure
: rewards and punishment
: nature and necessity of
feedback
And so on with   Aim Four – Ward Management
Aim Five – Personnel Management
Aim Six – Nursing Research

Table 1. Staff nurse development aims and learning objectives.

training in an authoritarian teaching environment that ill-prepares them for the dynamic responsibilities they have to face on the ward. Their further education has been conspicuously neglected. Now, when their demands for more training are being heard, the time is also right for them to collaborate in shaping their own further development.

Shifting into this mode of joint-responsibility requires a bit of a helping hand from those who have more experience and the will to show the way. Practical tools are also needed, like the guidelines given to participants, which show nurses how to start assessing themselves, start discussing their progress with other more senior people and making judgements for themselves on what to pursue for their own development.

The Hillingdon programme of self-development is supported by an off-the-job programme in which the nurses attend a five-day course with an emphasis on raising their self-awareness. This involves profiles, questionnaires and exercises which introduce them to different models and languages for understanding their thinking style and behavioural styles (Table 2). The nurses find the introduction to this approach exciting because for most of them psychology is a new world – and this approach involves the psychology of health and self-confidence through self-awareness, rather than the psychology of illness.

The 'B' Model (O'Neill, unpublished).
The Colours Model (Rhodes and Thame, 1988).
Transactional Analysis (Harris, 1973).
Temperaments Model for Stress (Thame, unpublished).
Maslow's Hierarchy of Needs (1954).
Theory X and Y (McGregor, 1960)
Hygiene and Motivation Factors (McGregor, 1960).

Table 2. Models used in the staff development programme.

Underlying the variety of approaches is a common thread – the unravelling of the processes of management and communication. The key to development, as we see it, is systems learning; recognising patterns within different kinds of data, so that knowledge from one situation can be transferred to the next. Although this is central to the nursing process, many nurses find it difficult to understand and apply. This is a special field of research and study by our consultancy (Rhodes and Thame, 1988), so our knowhow fitted well with the aims set out in the staff development programme.

Self-confidence

The first week of the programme devotes a lot of time to issues of self-confidence. On the fourth day there is a major exercise originally devised for salesmen, which involves a brain-storm in which the nurses generate lists of adjectives to describe their personalities to one another. They sort and categorise the listings into positive and negative attributes, based on observed behaviours during the course, then identify how each individual can work to capitalise on their strengths and improve on their weaknesses. Handling this kind of exercise must be done skillfully to ensure the individuals can work together honestly and supportively – its successful completion gives the nurses a real insight into the subtleties of self-assessment and leads to self-evaluation later in this programme.

The final day of the first week focuses on identifying key objectives for each nurse to work on. Although this is a detailed piece of work which involves considering many learning objectives, it is rewarding for the nurses because it sets the path for the kinds of tasks each must keep in the forefront of their mind. The week finishes with a visit to their new wards.

On-job learning

During their first months on the job the nurses are asked to keep a personal diary to encourage them in the processes of inner reflection. It is suggested that they write notes on their thoughts and feelings, what upsets them, what gives them pleasure, who they learn from, who makes difficulties, and so on. They are then asked to complete written assignments from the diaries, applying the behavioural models to real life happenings on the ward. This encourages them to look more objectively at situations which may have upset them at the time.

Throughout these weeks on the ward the nurses are visited and encouraged by the programme's nurse tutor, David Richards. Since this is David's first tutoring post, he has had to find his way, like the young nurses in the wards. This is especially exciting because it demonstrates the best qualities of joint development. David understands the ward situation, and his caring approach means the nurses have someone to turn to who knows the difficulties they face. At the same time, he can view their development not as their direct manager but indirectly, working with managers to enhance the nurses' learning opportunities.

Review and preparation for assignments

Our first study day, held in May 1988, produced encouraging developments. We began by reviewing the nurses' assignments, and heard some moving accounts of how they had tackled difficult situations using the behaviour models to help them analyse other people's intentions and shape their own responses. One particularly moving account told how one of the nurses encountered a desperately ill female patient who appeared to be showing aggression. Other nurses were struggling to restrain her, and the scene was violent and distressing. The nurse looked beyond the appearances, and recognised that the woman was terrified. A loving and calming hand was stretched out to her, soothed her and she became peaceful. A short while later she died. The nurse felt glad to have brought peace at the end.

The next activity was a series of role-plays through which the nurses could prepare for their next assignments. This involved their interviewing a senior member of staff to obtain information about a subject area they particularly wanted to investigate, linked to one of their learning objectives. For example, if they wished to extend their understanding of manpower management, they would interview a senior personnel officer. The nurses' first reactions were fear – they do not have much contact with senior people's roles, but after we had finished the role-plays they felt confident and excited at the prospects.

These assignments began in May 1988, and the first few months' progress caused great enthusiasm among the nurses. Later they attended the ENB 998 Teaching and Assessing course, and did a variety of assignments based around their six weekly off-the-job study days.

Developments since the programme's introduction

The nurses who joined the first programme have now graduated, and all plan to pursue their professional development through the Diploma in Nursing. The reports of their work have all been excellent and they have developed their confidence and skills in both practical nursing and communications.

This programme which commenced in March 1988 has run successfully, enabling 45 staff nurses to gain further development. However, due to the many changes in the NHS, our Health Authority and the education division, it has been necessary to discontinue the course in its present form with effect from March 1991.

All is not lost, though. Due to the noticeable benefits, the service side were very keen to continue with staff nurse development. Therefore a three month course commenced in September 1990 for Hillingdon Health Authority staff only. They are seconded from their area of appointment. We have maintained the same philosophy, aims and structure of the previous course. The course commences with a five day foundation and then five study days covering the same topics as in the previous course. The ENB 998 Teaching and Assessing in Clinical Practice has now been omitted.

References
Baker, B. (1987) *Guidelines of Course and Objectives.* Hillingdon Health Authority, London.
Harris, T. (1973) *I'm OK, Your OK.* Pan, London.
Herzberg, F. (1966) *Working and the Nature of Man.* World Publishing, Cleveland, Ohio.
McGregor, D. (1960) *The Human Side of Enterprise.* McGraw-Hill, New York.
Maslow, A.H. (1954) *Motivation and Personality.* Harper and Row, New York.
O'Neill, H. (Unpublished) *The 'B' Model.* Research for London Borough of Hillingdon.
Rhodes, J. and Thame, S. (1988) *The Colours of Your Mind.* Collins, London.
Rogers, J. and Lawrence, J. (1987) *Continuing Professional Education for Qualified Nurses, Midwives and Health Visitors.* Ashdale Press and Austen Cornish Publishers, London.
Thame, S. (Unpublished) Temperament Model For Stress.

Sue Thame, can be contacted at:
Sue Thame, Joint Development Resources,
24 Cecil Park, Pinner, Middx HA5 5HH.
Tel: 081-866 1262.

13

Teamwork: an equal partnership?

Gill Garrett, BA, SRN, RCNT, DN(Lond), CertEd(FE), RNT, FPCert
Freelance Lecturer, Bristol

From being one of the fundamental tenets in the care of groups such as elderly people and those with mental handicaps, the vital nature of the team approach has become recognised and accepted in all areas of nursing. Many patients have a multiplicity of needs – medical, nursing, therapeutic, social – which no one discipline can hope to meet; only by close collaboration and cooperation can different practitioners bring their skills into concert to attempt to meet them.

Increasingly in recent years, the validity of this contention has been appreciated by both hospital and community workers, and the gospel has been preached. But how effective has the concept been in practice? While no doubt in many parts of the country teams are working efficiently and harmoniously together to the benefit of all concerned, it would seem that in others there are areas of concern which demand urgent consideration and action if the concept is not to prove a meaningless cliché. With this in mind, we shall consider the prerequisites for effective teamwork, point out a few of the common problems which may arise and offer some suggestions as to how these problems may be ameliorated.

Who makes up the team?
One very basic question to ask before considering the work of the team is who makes up the team? On multiple choice papers, students will indicate the doctor, nurse, therapists, dietitians – all the professional partners in the venture. But integral to every team must be the people most meaningful to the individual patient: her family if she has any, her supportive neighbour, or whoever. If our aim is to rehabilitate the patient or to maintain her at her maximum level of functioning, these are people we neglect at our peril – and much more importantly, at the patient's peril. As professionals we must learn that we do not have a monopoly on care, nor do we have a dominant role in an unequal partnership. The contribution of relatives or friends, as agreeable to the patient, is vital – whether discussing assessments, setting goals or reviewing progress; their non-contribution, if excluded from active participation, may indeed frustrate all professional efforts. Although we shall

concentrate on those professionals who are conventionally seen as team members, this point cannot be overstressed.

Why are teams necessary?

Perhaps an even more basic question is, why does the team exist? It is easy to lose sight of the fact that its sole *raison d'être* is the patient and her need. An old adage runs, "The patient is the centre of the medical universe around which all our works revolve, towards which all our efforts trend". In economic terms we are quite used to this concept of 'consumer sovereignty', but in our health and social services management at present, all too often our consumer exists more to be 'done to' rather than canvassed for her opinion, offered options and helped to make choices. A thorny question often raised about the multidisciplinary team is, which professional should lead it? An equally important one not so often posed is, who should be the 'director' of team activity? If we recognise the patient as an autonomous, independent person (albeit with varying degrees of support), surely we must have the humility to acknowledge that this directing role falls inevitably to her. For patients with mental or other serious impairment, of course, the question of advocacy then arises – again an issue subject to much current debate.

Having allocated the role of director to the patient, the team leader then becomes the facilitator of action. It has been said that, "Fundamental to the concept of teamwork is . . . division of labour, coordination and task sharing, each member making a different contribution, but (one) of equal value, towards the common goal of patient care" (Ross, 1986). What do these elements demand? To make for efficient division of labour there has to be an accurate assessment of a situation and the input needed to deal with it, a recognition of who is the best person for which part of the job, and the carrying through of the appropriate allocation. Coordination demands the ability to see the overall, the sum of all the individual parts, and to recognise their relative weightings in various circumstances; it needs effective communication skills and the ability to use feedback to take adjustive action as required. Task-sharing demands that team members have an understanding of different roles and their effect upon one another, that they recognise areas of overlap and are prepared to shoulder one another's problems should the need arise. Such demands are not light; they require considerable training and practice to perfect.

Status and power within the team

Consideration of the second part of the Ross quotation brings us to one of the common problems experienced in multidisciplinary teamwork: ". . . of equal value towards the common goal of patient care". Is that how all team members view their own contribution or that of their partners? Status and power imbalances can make for great difficulties in team functioning; tradition accords high status and consequent power to the medical establishment, for example, with much affection but little standing to nurses. But if nurses have been seen as lacking in power and status, even lower on the rungs of the ladder comes the patient; in general, society grants a very low status to ill and disabled people, and institutional care strips all vestiges of power from inhabitants.

For workers who see themselves as being the juniors in teams, the presence and influence of more powerful members may prove intimidating, and consequently they may make only tentative and limited contributions to discussions and meetings. It is important that they realise that, however 'junior', they have a right to contribute, indeed a duty to do so, if they have what has been described as the "authority of relevance" (Webb and Hobdell, 1975) – if they have knowledge relevant to the patient's own feelings of need or wellbeing which must be brought to the team's attention. So often it is those members who spend more time in close proximity to the patient who possess such authority, rather than the senior medical personnel who may visit her only on a weekly basis.

'Follow my leader'   A second problem may arise out of the power and status imbalance, especially when team members have become used to suppressing their views or do not recognise their authority of relevance – regression into the 'follow my leader' phenomenon. There may be the tendency to leave all the thinking to another group member who is perceived as being more prestigious or simply more articulate, often the consultant. His thinking and directions are seen as definitive, with team members abdicating their own professional responsibility to think and speak for themselves and for their patient from their own vantage points. Except in the unlikely event of the team leader being qualified in a multidisciplinary capacity, this obviously acts to the detriment of patient care – we can none of us prescribe or wholly substitute for each other's contributions. A variation on this 'follow my leader' phenomenon is sometimes seen where two leaders emerge from subgroups in a team, each with his or her own following. In addition to the drawbacks already mentioned, the results in situations like this are invariably divisive too.

'Groupthink'   This is the name that has been given to another possible problem in teamwork; it is generally seen in well-established, long-lived teams whose members over time have grown very used to working with each other. Team meetings are always amicable and 'cosy', there is no bickering or dissension and everyone gets on terribly well with everyone else. The group gives the appearance of having its own internal strength, with a marked sense of loyalty and supportiveness. But this denies that disagreement and conflict are facts of life and often signs of constructive enquiry and growth; all too often such teams ". . . become rigid, committed to the status quo . . . less open to input and feedback.

Hierarchies become established and bureaucratic qualities emerge which resist questioning and change" (Brill, 1976).

Patient confusion   In case this should all seem a little esoteric, consider for a moment one last very basic possible problem in multidisciplinary teamwork – potential confusion for the patient. Unless each member of the team extends to her the courtesy of an introduction to their personal role, with an explanation of how this fits in with the overall individual plan of care, especially in the acute phase of an illness, the patient (particularly if elderly) may well find so many professionals overwhelming and muddling. If she is to feel in any degree in control of the situation and if any confusion is to be lessened, time must be taken to ensure a personal approach, with all care being presented as part of a concerted whole, and with common goals identified towards which all the team are working.

This last problem, then, is usually amenable to a common courtesy and common sense solution. But what about the others? The problems associated with status and 'follow my leader' have a more deep-seated origin and, although rectifiable in the short term in individual teams, in the longer term they demand a close scrutiny of, and changes in, professional education. 'Groupthink' demands flexibility of individuals and a system which encourages and permits a regular turnover of personnel to maintain healthy group dynamics.

Common core training?

If in effective teams there is no room for professional superiorities or jealousies, what is needed is an open, trusting relationship based on knowledge of, and respect for, one another's professional expertise. But this demands in turn an insight into other trainings and backgrounds to understand one another's terms of reference – the differences in emphasis we have in relation to patient care. While individual effort and inservice training programmes can go some way towards this, the difficulties with late attitudinal change are only too well known. Most of our basic feelings about our own profession and those with which we work are formed during our initial training period. Nursing is currently implementing Project 2000, with a common core foundation programme for all nurse practitioners. Is it not time we were much more adventurous, and explored avenues of common core training for all health professionals? Certain knowledge, skills and attitudes are prerequisites whether we are to be doctors, nurses, therapists or social workers – if we learned them together how much easier it would be to practise them together. The intention of such common training would not be to reduce all teaching to the lowest common denominator, but rather to look at areas of mutual concern, highlighting the unique contribution of each professional, and the bearing this has on the work of the other team members.

Value of difference

Educational change may also help us to recognise the value of 'difference' and the constructive use to which conflict may be put, so that 'groupthink' becomes a less likely problem. Better training in interpersonal skills – including assertiveness – should help the creation of a climate in which there is freedom to differ, to look more dispassionately at dissent, while acknowledging the areas of basic trust and agreement that do exist and can be built upon. The need for turnover in team membership has to be balanced, of course, by the need for reasonable stability over a period of time. Change every five minutes for the sake of it helps no one, but there must be recognition that long-term team stagnation (however well camouflaged) is beneficial neither to the group nor to the professionals within it – and certainly not to the patient and her family.

Realism

This chapter provides only a brief overview of a very important area. Readers' personal experiences may differ considerably from the scenarios which have been outlined. It would seem, however, that most experienced nurses have had the experience of needing to temper idealism in striving for effective teamwork with realism, given the situations in which they work. But recognition of this is in itself a step forward; we must have in mind that "under the aegis of teamwork, strange bedfellows are discovering, in time, that they must *learn* to work together before they *can* work together . . . teamwork is not an easy process to understand or to practise" (Brill, 1976).

References

Brill, N.I. (1976) *Teamwork: Working Together in the Human Services*. Lippincott, New York.
Ross, F.M. (1986) Nursing old people in the community. In: Redfern, S. (ed) *Nursing Elderly People*. Churchill Livingstone, Edinburgh.
Webb, A.L. and Hobdell, M. (1975) Coordination between health and personal social services: a question of quality. In: Interaction of social welfare and health personnel in the delivery of services: Implications for training. Eurosound Report No. 4, Vienna.

14
Making the team work!

John Øvretveit, C.Psychol, BSc, MPhil, DPhil
Co-Director, Health Services Centre, Institute of Organisation and Social Studies,
Brunel University

Multidisciplinary community teams are often seen as the cornerstone of
specialist services in the community for such client groups as people
with mental health problems, learning difficulties, addiction problems
and elderly people with special needs. It is therefore surprising that, for
the most part, little thought and preparation has been given to how they
will operate. We shall outline here those features which are essential to
the continued success of any team, irrespective of the personalities, aims
or organisations involved.

Research method
This chapter draws on a continuing programme of collaborative field
research initiated in 1984 with a variety of teams and managers in
England and Wales (Øvretveit, 1986) using two types of research:
- Long-term collaboration with individual teams on particular problems
  of team organisation. The teams are helped to describe features of their
  current organisation and to clarify alternative future options eg, for
  referral, case records and crisis services. The team and their managers
  agree and operate the new arrangement, and the researcher monitors
  its effectiveness. Two three-year projects of this type were undertaken
  (Macdonald and Øvretveit, 1987; Macdonald, 1989).
- Other research data comes from problem-centred two-day workshops
  for teams wishing to improve their organisation or for health and
  social services managers wishing to develop teams. Two common
  types of workshops were: to set up new teams in other areas of a
  district, learning from others already set up, and to help members of a
  team which is not working well to collaborate more closely.

In a number of cases follow-up workshops were held, to ascertain
whether the solutions actually worked. To date 68 of these workshops
have been held across the UK, and the research has found that three
ingredients are essential to the success of any team: a common base, a
team leader and an operational policy. However, we need to be clear why
a multidisciplinary team is necessary before we can consider which type
of team is most suitable. Given the problems and expense involved in
setting up a successful team, both members and managers need to be
convinced the advantages are worth the time and effort involved.

Advantages of multiprofessional teams

Why should professional practitioners with different training and perspectives and from different agencies, work closely together in teams? The advantages of multidisciplinary teams are listed below.

Better service   The main function of multidisciplinary teams is to ensure clients get a better service than they would otherwise receive from independent professional and agency help. Although agencies and professionals can agree arrangements for certain professionals to act as case-coordinators, it is usually better if case-coordinators are part of a permanent team. Case-coordinators have an agreed role and are allocated cases through the team. In this way, the team acts as the clear point for all referrals, and clients can rely on one familiar person to help in dealing with the bewildering bureaucracy and range of services they need. By working in a multidisciplinary team, case-coordinators have immediate access to a range of professionals and agencies, and develop a better understanding of the special skills and resources each has to offer, making them better able to meet the needs of clients.

Specialist practitioners working together can identify gaps in local services and formulate proposals for improvements based on understanding and experience of local client needs. It is easier for practitioners to plan and run projects as a team than individually.

Easier workload management   Teams also make it easier to manage workload and to establish common priorities across professions. For teams to work, each profession and agency must agree whether its practitioners will participate part- or full-time. This ensures a stable resource of specialists for the client group. Given the time and skills available, difficult decisions have to be made about priorities, but teams do allow practitioners to share work, with each member undertaking a fair share of unpopular as well as popular work.

Colleague support   Practitioners can often receive vital support and advice from other team members in dealing with complex cases. For example, some community mental handicap nurses are managed by a general community nurse manager, but find a senior social worker in mental handicap understands more than their manager about problems they have with particular clients and their families. Of course, certain types of technical advice can only come from a member of the same profession, and regular contact is necessary to keep up-to-date in profession-specific skills and knowledge. Emotional support is also important in stressful work with clients, and members can be of great help to each other in the team.

The benefits of teamwork do not come about simply because managers and planning groups call a group of practitioners a 'team'. Teams must be planned, funded, nurtured and regularly reviewed. Managers and team members must be clear what type of team they are establishing, and why it is the best arrangement for their client group.

Types of team

Table 1 describes five different types of team. This distinction is the first step in deciding which type of team is necessary. All too often, planning groups recommend a multidisciplinary team be set up without seriously considering which type is most appropriate or whether a team is required at all. Given the time, expense and problems involved in setting up a successful team, managers need to be convinced that such a service is the best way of using scarce resources to meet needs. Unfortunately, there is little objective evidence on the effectiveness of different types of team in different circumstances, and managers need to seek out the experience of others to find what has and has not worked.

The starting point should be an objective and systematic assessment of client needs and the resources available. However, it is usually only after it has been set up that the team begins to look more closely at how it is organised, and develops an accurate assessment of its needs and resources. The five models help clarify how a team is and should be organised.

Clarifying the team leader role

If a decision is made that 'closer' teamwork is required, attention should be given to agreeing common catchment areas for each profession, defining the time allocated by each member to teamwork and establishing a single base. In addition, it is necessary to channel all referrals to this base to establish the identity of the team, to clarify the team leader role and detail an operational policy. The following describes some essentials for establishing accountable service-delivery teams.

The quickest way to establish close and effective teamwork is to start with a clearly defined team leader role. I do not know of any teams which have close teamwork and have survived changes of membership without a clear team leader position. One of the biggest mistakes is to believe that interprofessional and interagency conflicts, rivalries and protectionism can be avoided by not defining a team leader role. Managers cause more conflict and bad feeling in the long run by encouraging the idea that leaving things ambiguous gives them more room to maneouvre in future. It is better to face up to differences and agree the role before problems arise, and recrimination or mistrust result.

Even so-called 'democratic teams' have leaders for different functions, recognising that agreed authority is required to get things done. The main issue is which type of team leader to appoint. This depends on the work they are responsible for, who they are accountable to and the sanctioned authority they have over team members.

A useful way to clarify the division of responsibilities and authority between the team leader and the professional superior is to consider each

Profession-managed informal network One arrangement, sometimes described as a team, is where each practitioner remains under the management of their professional manager but takes part in regular meetings with other practitioners working with the same client group in the same area. Usually no-one is required to attend or is bound to the 'decisions' made at the meeting, and there is no collective responsibility for providing a combined service. The meetings arise out of the common interests of practitioners in the same area for information exchange, to improve cross-referrals and, on occasion, to arrange shared projects.

Fully-managed multidisciplinary team Teams with *one* full manager accountable for each practitioner's work and for the service provided by the team. The manager has authority to appoint, assign work, appraise performance and to discipline members. The team usually works on consensus, but with the awareness that final accountability and authority rests with the team manager. In the past, some psychiatric teams operated in this way, and in the US some psychiatric clinics follow this model. The modern variant usually involves a nominated professional advisor outside the team giving advice on aspects of the team members' practice, management, professional training and development.

Coordinated team with shared management A more common arrangement where each profession (and agency) endorses the role of a team coordinator, who shares responsibilities for managing team members with professional superiors outside the team. The team coordinator is appointed by higher management and is accountable to them for coordinating team members. He or she may, however, be nominated from among the team. Team coordinators rarely have authority to review or override profession-specific case decisions of senior practitioners, but often participate in aspects of management such as appointment and appraisal. Many community mental handicap teams in Wales use this model, with a social services appointee as coordinator.

Core and extended team This term is used to describe at least two types of team. In one, the core team consists of full-time members (usually nurses and/or social workers), and the extended team of part-time members, usually covering a wider area (such as psychiatrists, clinical psychologists, occupational therapists and speech therapists). In the second type, the core team is directly managed by the team leader who coordinates the extended team which often works elsewhere (for example, a core team of psychiatric nurses based in a day hospital and managed by a community psychiatric nurse manager who also coordinates social workers and other therapists).

'Joint accountability' or 'democratic team' In these teams, there is no team leader although there may be a team 'secretary' appointed by and accountable to the team. Depending on the task, the team will agree that one member carries out a leadership role for a particular task, with authority delegated by the team meeting. If consensus cannot be reached on a particular issue, the team will use an agreed procedure (usually majority vote) to reach a binding decision. However, majority vote cannot override a member's profession-specific responsibilities.

Table 1. The types of team.

of the areas of personnel management in Table 2 and establish individual or joint responsibility for each task. It is usually possible to define the rights and authority of the two roles by the following three types of authority (Table 3). There are a number of arguments for assigning full responsibility and authority to the team leader, with professional superiors in an 'advisory' role. Members are then challenged to explain the problems which can occur in both the short and long term. Research has found that if the professional superior retains the right to allocate work (management task 3, authority C), this restricts the time a member is available for teamwork and limits the closeness of teamwork possible.

1. Draft job description. 2. Shortlist, interview and appoint. 3. Assign cases and work. 4. Review cases and work. 5. Annual performance appraisal. 6. Training. 7. Disciplinary matters.

Table 2. Areas in which responsibility should be established between the team leader and professional superior.

A The right to be informed or consulted. Should, for example, a community psychiatric nurse manager consult with a team leader (who may be a social worker) about the appointment of a community mental health nurse? **B** Joint decision (both team leader and professional superior have the right to veto). Following the above example, should the team leader have the right to veto the appointment? **C** The right to decide. Should the nurse manager have the ultimate decision, with or without consulting the team leader?

Table 3. Three types of authority which should be specified between team leader and professional superior.

Operational policy

One of the most important tasks of a team leader is to regularly review the operational policy or to formulate one to propose if management has not provided one. The operational policy is the team leader's main working tool, authorising him or her to call for changes if members do not follow agreed ways of working.

Teams often do not specify the referral procedure to be followed by its members. In one situation, a team leader found that a nurse could not take a priority case referred to the team, which only a nurse could deal with. It emerged that the nurse's caseload was full with cases she had been taking independently from GPs and from a psychiatrist in another area. The team leader assumed all cases went through the team; this was not, however, agreed policy and the team leader had no authority to alter the nurse's practice to ensure the priority case was allocated.

To be a team, is by definition, to have an operational policy: group members need agreements about who will do what in different situations. The only issue is whether the policy is explicit or implicit, in the degree of detail and the areas covered. The advantages of explicit policy are that members are clear about agreed ways of working; it offers guidance; it explains and publicises the purpose and organisation of the team and enables it to monitor and improve its organisation.

A good starting point for a team establishing its policy is to write down their arrangements under certain headings, before discussing and agreeing improvements. The list of headings in Table 4 has proved useful to a number of teams beginning to detail or review their policy.

There are a number of ways of meeting the special needs of people living in the community. It has often been thought necessary to provide more specialist help in the community, and to improve collaboration between professionals. Multidisciplinary community teams have been viewed as the main method of improving services, but usually little thought is given to which type of team is appropriate. If 'close' teamwork is required, a common base which acts as the focal point for referrals is necessary. The role of team leader and team operational policy

---

Aims, priorities, client group and catchment area General purpose of the team, definition of client groups served by the team and those which are not, boundaries of catchment area.

Team philosophy, objectives and priorities General principles informing members of the work and the services offered by the team; specific objectives and current ordering of priorities.

Team membership Name, profession and role, special skills, time available for 'team work' and contact point.

Referrals to and from the team Criteria for accepting assessment and long-term work as a 'team responsibility'; criteria for finishing team involvement; arrangements for informing referrer of actions.

Team meetings   Conduct, agendas and decision-making procedures for team casework decisions, for team management and policy decisions, and for team proposals for service developments.

Case allocation, case-coordination and cross-referrals How cases are allocated for assessment and long-term work; responsibilities of case-coordinator; how cross-referrals and co-working within the team is arranged.

Team leader role Responsibilities; accountability; authority; method of appointment.

Professional superior roles Responsibilities; accountability; authority of each professional superior in and out of the team.

Team systems and procedures General heading eg, for workload statistics and information systems, case records and client access policy, finance and budgets, complaints procedure, staff performance appraisal and development.

Team accountability and performance reporting Group or individual to whom the team is responsible, and their responsibilities to the team; frequency and nature of team reports of workload, achievements and difficulties.

Appendices Proposals for service developments and update plans.

Table 4. Issues to consider in planning or reviewing team policy.

also need to be detailed, agreed and sanctioned. If thought is given to the general framework within which the team is to work, members can concentrate on the details of how they will work together.

References

MacDonald, I. (Ed) (1987) *Managing Change in a Mental Handicap Hospital.* Mental Handicap Services Unit, Brunel University.

MacDonald, I. (Ed) (1989) *The Rhondda Vanguard Community Mental Handicap Service.* Mental Handicap Service Unit, Working Paper, Brunel University.

Øvretveit, J. (1986) *Management and Democratic Teams.* BPS, Clinical Psychology Forum, October.

Øvretveit, J. (1986) *Organising Multidisciplinary Community Teams.* HSC Working Paper, BIOSS, Brunel University.

Øvretveit, J. (1987) Aspects of CMHT Organisation and Management. In: Grant, Humphreys and McGrath (Eds) *Community Mental Handicap Teams: Theory and Practice.* British Institute of Mental Handicap, Kidderminster, Worcs.

15

Promoting self-directed enquiry

Janice Hoover, RNT, BScN, RN, SRN

Lecturer in Advanced Nursing, South Glamorgan School of Nursing

Much of student nurses' learning is passive, the mere ingestion of facts to be regurgitated at a later date to obtain a grade in an exam. It is not uncommon to hear student nurses asking qualified nurses to impart their textbook knowledge to them: "Teach me about congestive cardiac failure". How do nurses learn and develop once they become qualified, when to ask such questions is unacceptable? Besides, who would the qualified nurse ask?

Nursing care conferences

In March, 1986, at a study day organised by the King's Fund Centre in London, my nurse manager, ward nursing tutor and myself (a ward sister) were asked as a 'triad' from Llandough Hospital, South Glamorgan Health Authority, to consider one aspect of 'The developing role of the ward sister'. Interested in attacking this problem of passivity in nurse learning and in finding a way to encourage staff members to assist themselves to learn, we chose to examine the ward sister's role as an educator. So we began the 'nursing care conferences' on our ward (an acute 30-bed medical/geriatric ward).

In 1968, Knowles coined the word "andragogy" to describe an emerging science of adult learning. The greatest learning experiences are believed to result from methods which involve the learner intensely in self-directed enquiry. Adult learning is thought to be a process which occurs *within* the individual (Rosendahl, 1974).

The educator does not merely transmit knowledge, but facilitates another person's learning through self-directed enquiry. This is what we set out to achieve, with the nursing care conferences.

It was planned to ask a qualified nurse or two or three learners to present a nursing article, nursing care plan or topic of nursing interest to the rest of the ward nursing team for group consideration and discussion. Each presentation was to last from 30 to 40 minutes. We hoped that this would be a first step towards stimulating a life long habit of self-directed enquiry.

We devised a questionnaire to measure nurses' attitudes and behaviour related to the self-directed learning process. We wanted to measure these variables before and after participation in the project to determine the project's success and, to discover any correlation between different nursing grades and initiative in self-learning. However, due to our questionnaire's small sample size, we felt that to do so would have threatened the anonymity of everyone completing the questionnaire. Also, any correlation which we might have found using such a small sample would not have been particularly significant. The pre-project questionnaire results, however, did provide us with the ward nurses' overall support for our project. Most were "keen" or "very keen" to participate and thought that they would learn more by presenting a topic for discussion rather than by listening to topics presented by others.

Enabling change

Change, no matter how well supported, can lead to staff resistance, so we attempted to establish as much favour for the project as possible. The following techniques (New and Couillard, 1981) were used:

Education   Six weeks before the project started, it was explained to staff that a great deal could be learned by sharing their different nursing interests, knowledge and experience with each other. Current good patient care on the ward could only stand to improve further from such an exchange. It was also explained in detail how the project was to be implemented and what would be expected of both the presenters and the rest of the group.

Gradual introduction   Introducing the project well in advance, gave the staff time and opportunity to realise the benefits of the change. The ward sister presented the first conference to demonstrate what was expected. They were to be held once a fortnight to allow individuals time to adapt to the idea. Each nurse would be given her presentation date at least one month in advance to give her time to prepare.

Supportive behaviour   To assist anyone with any difficulties in selecting or presenting their topic of interest, the ward sister offered herself as a resource person (with the stipulation that she be given 'reasonable' notification of any help required). It was stressed that the project is not a competition though it is hoped that individuals will be spurred on by each others interesting presentations to do their best.

Incentives   With a schedule of fortnightly conferences, each individual would be called on to present a topic approximately only once every eight months. It was stressed that the rest of the time one would be free to enjoy listening to others' presentations.

Participation   While the design and implementation of the project had already been decided, an enthusiastic senior staff nurse was asked to promote the most positive aspects of the project to the others.

Two further techniques were employed to lessen resistance to change. First, the more enthusiastic individuals were selected to present topics first in the hope that they might generate enthusiasm in the others. Second, high expectations of the presentations going ahead as scheduled were set by the ward sister. Postponements because of difficulties in completing work on time were not considered without a strong suggestion that more efficient organisation of time could get the job done. It was hoped that if people were tacitly 'expected' to complete a task, they would feel an onus on them to do so.

Once the nursing care conferences began in July, 1986, it became the ward sister's responsibility to ask the group questions and to stimulate thoughtful creative discussion relevant to the group's area of practice (Plummer, 1974).

This focusing on the specific problems of everyday practice is vital in making the conferences interesting and valuable as a learning experience for everyone. Praise and encouragement are given to presenters and the non-presenters when merited to reinforce individuals' positive feelings about themselves and their abilities and accomplishments. It is not yet possible to measure the project's success because not everyone has presented their first topic.

Staff perceptions

More than half the nurses (of all grades) have commented that they think that the conferences are a good idea, in that they helped to keep them up-to-date. They view this as very important and, are keen to apply new knowledge which they acquire from the sessions. The more relevant and interesting they perceive the topics and related discussions to be, the more actively and enthusiastically they participate in the conferences.

Motivation

The conferences have provided the motivating environment now thought necessary for learning (Gordon, 1982). They are a channel, through which individual enquiry (coupled with group discussion) into topics of each individual's own nursing interests is directed. With the ward sister's help as a conference leader, staff confidence in presenting their findings to the rest of the ward nursing team has expanded. Staff development and education have been facilitated with minimal extra resources and it is hoped that a broad foundation has been laid for a life-time of learning.

References

Gordon, G.K. (1982) Motivating staff: A look at assumptions. *The Journal of Nursing Administration*, **12**, 11, 28.

New, J.R. et al, (1981) Guidelines for introducing change: *The Journal of Nursing Administration*, **11**, 3, 18–20.

Plummer, E.M. (1974) The clinical conference discussion leader. *Nursing Forum*, 13, 1, 94 and 103.

Rosendahl, P. (1974) Self-direction for learners: an andragogical approach to nursing education. *Nursing Forum*, **13**, 2, 138.

Bibliography
United Kingdom Central council for Nursing Midwifery and Health Visiting, Educational Policy Advisory Committee, (1986) *Project 2000, A New Preparation for Practice.*
Proposals for the education of nurses in Great Britain by the year 2000.

16

Negligence: defining responsibility

David Carson, LLB
Senior Lecturer, Faculty of Law, University of Southampton

The six tests

When dealing with cases of alleged negligence in nursing, the courts do not just ask "Was the behaviour negligent?" They go through a series of separate tests which, together, make up the law of negligence. It is most easily understood as six questions.

1. Did the nurse owe a duty of care to the injured person?
2. Did the nurse break the appropriate standard of care in the circumstances?
3. Did that breach of the standard cause the injuries?
4. Are the injuries of a kind that the courts compensate?
5. Were the injuries reasonably forseeable?
6. Did the injured person contribute to the happening of, or the extent of, the injuries?

Questions 1 to 5 must be answered "Yes." If not there is no legal liability. If question 6 is answered "Yes" then there has been contributory negligence, which means that the injured person's compensation will be reduced.

Court decisions are illustrative but it is dangerous to generalise from the facts rather than the law. Injecting a patient in the wrong place may break the standard of care in one case but not in another where, for example, there are special reasons such as an emergency.

The duty of care

Nurses only owe a duty of care to certain people, certainly to their patients and colleagues. But how do the courts decide who else nurses legally owe a duty of care? In *Towers v. Cambridgeshire Area Health Authority & Others* (unreported, March 9, 1982) an ambulanceman injured his back lifting a heavy patient. Anticipating a difficult lift, his colleague asked, two or three times, for help. One nurse took a drip but otherwise his requests were ignored. They began to lift. The colleague lost his grip and Mr Towers had to take the patient's weight. His back was injured.

Did the nurses owe the ambulance officers a duty of care? The trial judge said that nurses were not "primarily carriers" and there might be other claims upon their attention. So it did not matter how unreasonable or bad the nurses' behaviour was; they were not liable because they had no duty of care to the ambulance officers. The Court of Appeal disagreed. The trial judge had confused the second question about the standard of care with the first question about the duty of care. If a nurse had something more important to do then he or she would not be in breach of the *standard* but could still owe a *duty* of care to the ambulance officer.

The courts say we owe duties of care to our 'neighbours', people whom it is reasonably foreseeable may be affected by our actions and inactions. On this occasion it was reasonably foreseeable that these ambulance officers would have been affected by these nurses' behaviour. It may not be possible to imagine some of the people nurses owe duties to. Discharge a patient early and the relatives may harm themselves in trying to cope. Is that reasonably foreseeable? Is it reasonably foreseeable that a head injury patient will suffer further if not told to seek immediate attention if he or she begins to vomit? Many things are foreseeable. But it must be reasonable, not fanciful.

The standard of care

The judges decide who is owed a duty of care but the profession invariably decides the standard of care. The essential question is whether the nurse acted in a way that reasonably competent nurses would have done in those circumstances?

In *Walker v. South West Surrey D.H.A.* (unreported, June 17, 1982) a woman was giving birth. She said that she was injected with pethidine in the inner side of her right thigh. That fact was disputed, though both sides agreed that if it was true then it broke the standard of care. ''No careful nurse or doctor would give an injection at that point unless there was some compelling reason to do so.''

The standard is not what the best nurse or what most nurses or the average nurse would have done. It is about the reasonably competent nurse in that, if any, specialty. Expert witnesses may be called. They will be asked whether reasonably competent nurses would have done that. The test is not what the witness would have done. The test depends upon and reinforces professional standards. Certainly the courts reserve the right to declare professional practices and standards too low but that is a rarely applied reserve power.

The test recognises that standards should keep improving. What was reasonably competent once, say not knowing about adverse reactions to a new drug, will soon become unreasonable. The role of journals in spreading information about new standards can be crucial. Failure to read a journal could be the breach of standard.

''The test is the standard of the ordinary skilled man exercising and professing to have that skill. A man need not possess the highest expert skill: it is well established law that it is sufficient if he exercises the ordinary skill of an ordinary competent man exercising that particular art.'' That is known as the *Bolam* test. *(Bolam v. Friern H.M.C.* [1957] 1 W.L.R. 582,

586.) It has been restated many times by many courts. While it involved a doctor, the same principles would apply to a nurse. The test recognises differences of professional opinion. Provided a responsible body of professional opinion would support the action, the standard is met. Without differences of opinion there is no progress.

Causation

A patient in a psychiatric hospital had florid delusions about Christ, snakes, fires and said she had to die. She was diagnosed as having a "depressive illness with some paranoid features". She was to be nursed on the ward but not subjected to constant observation. She was noted as being potentially suicidal and likely to abscond. One day her husband gave a nurse a box of matches. He explained that his wife had given them to him saying that she might otherwise set fire to herself. This was not noted in the nursing records. The patient had periods of being very disturbed, shouted about fires, escaped from the ward but returned voluntarily. Her consultant concluded that she was in a psychotic state. He did not alter the nursing instructions. Then one day she seemed calmer, agreed to join in some activities but first went to the toilet, alone. There she set fire to her tee-shirt and burnt herself badly.

The patient claimed that both the doctors and the nurse were negligent. The doctors should have required constant observation. The nurse ought to have recorded the incident with the box of matches. The trial judge decided that the doctors were not negligent; reasonably competent doctors in that position would not have required constant observation. The matchbox incident, however, should have been recorded. Thus the nurse owed a duty of care to the patient and the standard of care had been broken. The nurse was therefore negligent, the trial court decided.

The Court of Appeal disagreed. (*Gauntlett v. Northampton Health Authority*, unreported, December 12, 1985.) The trial judge had confused the separate questions about breach of the standard of care and causation. The evidence was that if the consultant had known of the matchbox incident he would still not have required constant observation. The injuries would still have happened. The nurse may have behaved improperly but that did not cause the injuries. Many would link the matchbox incident and the subsequent burning but it is the effect on the decision-makers that counts; ". . professional experience of dealing with people with disordered minds gives it a much less literal significance, as an indication of possible, or probable, future acts by the patient."

The causation rule in the law of negligence requires us to think twice. If the injuries would have happened anyway then some apparent causes might not be causes at all. (But disciplinary action could still be taken for the breach of the standard of care which, luckily, did not cause injury.) But this point must not be overstated. That several people cause somebody's injuries simply means that each is liable and the court will settle how much each should pay.

If the injuries would still have happened, but not so soon or so extensively, then those have been caused. In *Sutton v. Population Services Planning Programme Ltd.* (unreported, October 31, 1981) a nurse was working in a well-woman centre. When a patient complained of a lump in a breast she was supposed, it was agreed, to refer her to a doctor at the centre. She did not, and the patient subsequently had a mastectomy. Thus there was a duty of care and a breach of the standard of care. But, it was accepted, the doctor would not have found the lump, even with a mammograph. Did the nurse's breach cause the loss? The Court examined the steps likely to have been taken. The doctor would have referred to a specialist. The specialist would not have found anything but told the GP. The patient would have returned and repeated her complaint. The GP would have sent her to a specialist. The specialist would have found the lump, with or without a mammograph, and operated a few days later. The operation would have taken place about 10 weeks before it actually did take place and caught the cancer at an early stage. The patient would then have had a greater chance of survival for longer. Thus the nurse's breach of the proper standard did cause the loss.

Foreseeable losses
The courts will only compensate certain kinds of loss. This certainly includes injuries to the person and their finances. Pain, suffering and loss of amenities are covered. They will compensate recognised psychiatric disorders but are reluctant to compensate experiences such as sorrow and upset and not just because of problems of proof.

Recognised loss
A recognised loss or injury might nevertheless go uncompensated because the way it occurred was not reasonably foreseeable. This point is unlikely to arise frequently in nursing cases but it is possible. Say a mentally disordered patient leaves a hospital, through a nurse's breach of standard of care, and causes problems for a relative. Presuming the nurse owes a duty of care to the relative, he or she is unlikely to be liable if the loss or injury was, for example, to the relative's investment portfolio. That could be regarded as not reasonably foreseeable.

Contributory negligence
It is the plaintiff, the patient, who might be guilty of contributory negligence. If he or she is guilty, then the compensation will be reduced by the proportion by which the court thinks he or she is to blame. It includes both contributing to the cause or happening of the accident and contributing to the amount or extent of the injuries or losses by, for example, not seeking medical attention or disregarding advice. In *Patel v. Adyha* (unreported, April 2, 1985) a patient consulted her GP about back pains. His examination broke the standard of care. He should have discovered symptoms which would have led him to refer the patient to

a specialist who would have diagnosed a tubercular condition with kyphosis. She deteriorated and, according to the judgement, her spine 'collapsed'. The doctor's lawyer argued that she should have sought further medical attention when her problems would have been noted and treated in time. But the Court of Appeal decided that it was perfectly understandable that she did not return to her doctor when she had been led to believe that there was nothing that could be done. However, if she had been "inviting disaster," if she had not acted as a reasonable person in her condition would have acted then, the Court implied, she would have been contributorily negligent.

17

Taking risks with patients: your assessment strategy

David Carson, LLB
Senior Lecturer, Faculty of Law, University of Southampton

Nurses make judgements, decisions. Nurses take risks. An elderly patient may be allowed matches in his bed despite the risk of fire. A mentally disordered patient may commit suicide while allowed the freedom of the hospital grounds. A patient discharged early may be unable to cope. There is a dignity and individuality in being able and allowed to take risks. In fact, taking risks is often a highly valued activity. But, despite the hope for and expectation of success, there is a risk of harm for the patient – and a risk of litigation, disciplinary action or professional inquiry for the nurse. Although risks may be frightening and worrying, risk-taking can be the essence of professional responsibility. Here we will outline a way of assessing risks. It encourages risk-taking after careful analysis of the risk and, properly used, should prevent legal liability and professional censure if things should go wrong.

Making decisions

The method outlined below describes an approach to risk-taking. It does not take the decision away from nurses, nor provide easy solutions for individual cases. It does not tell nurses *what* to decide, rather it suggests a *way* of deciding. In view of the increasing pressure on resources and new care philosophies which encourage risk-taking and patients' rights, this framework could help in making decisions. Indeed, it might be used as the basis of a risk-taking policy which health authorities could adopt with a promise to support those staff who follow it. The framework is as follows:

1. Analyse whether the proposed action is best described as a gamble, a risk or a dilemma.

2. List all the possible kinds of benefits, for the patient, of acting.

3. List all the possible kinds of benefits, and knock-on benefits, for other people.

4. Analyse the likelihood of each of these benefits occurring.

5. Manipulate the risk by taking steps to make the benefits more likely

to occur.

6. List all the possible kinds of harm, to the patient, of acting.

7. List all the possible kinds of harm, and knock-on harms, to other people.

8. Analyse the likelihood of each of these harms occurring.

9. Manipulate the risk by taking steps to reduce the likelihood of the harms occurring.

10. List any duties to risk.

11. Obtain the patient's informed consent.

12. Obtain the informed agreement of colleagues.

13. Assess whether 'the risk' should be taken.

Gamble, risk or dilemma?

Consider three different activities; gambling, taking a risk and facing up to a dilemma. Which is it that nurses do? Gambling is something that *may* be done (it does not have to be done) to gain a benefit where the act of gambling is often pleasurable. Taking risks involves deciding that the potential benefits of a proposed act outweigh the potential drawbacks. You may take risks because the potential benefits make it desirable. In contrast, facing a dilemma involves *having to act*, having to choose between options – each of which carries both potential benefits and potential harm. When facing a dilemma, something has to be done; doing nothing is, or soon will be, harmful.

Nurses' actions will often be better described as facing up to a dilemma rather than taking a risk. Merely calling it risk-taking is a disservice to both the nurses and their judges. Besides giving more credit and greater respect, we expect less and apply a lower standard when we know that a dilemma is involved. A situation requires quick thinking and action in the face of a dilemma. Who would argue with the questions: "We took a risk; can you say our decision was wrong?" and "We faced a dilemma; can you say our decision was wrong?"

Analysing decisions into gambles, risks and dilemmas is being truthful and honest, and fair judgements can be made. However, 'risk-taking' will be referred to here to avoid being repetitive.

The two sides to a risk

A risk can be divided into the *consequence* – the gain or loss, the benefit or injury that might occur – and the *likelihood* – the odds, the chance, the possibility, that it might occur. For example, there is a 10:1 risk (likelihood) the horse will win. There is a risk (consequence) I might lose £10 and a risk (consequence) I might win £100. Both senses of the word should be considered.

When the risk is of a dramatic injury or loss, like a patient's death or lifelong paralysis, we – quite naturally – get worried. But that is only one part of the risk. It is very easy to suggest that death is possible; it is possible every time we cross a road. A proper analysis of risk must consider the likelihood of each suggested outcome. A risk-taking scheme should ensure that the likelihood of each possible outcome is assessed separately. Epidemiological data may sometimes be used to describe statistically the chance but, if unavailable, words and concepts of possibility can be used. Precision may be impossible but that does not prevent clear thinking.

Benefits and losses

Another understandable tendency when taking risks is to concentrate on harms, injuries and losses. We tend to stress what may go wrong rather than what may succeed. When a child is returned from local authority care to its parents who then abuse it again, the press and media will concentrate on the risk of such abuse occurring. Little attention will be paid to the reasons for taking that risk, to the objectives of the exercise. However, if the decision was actually taken in terms of 'seeing if we can get away with it', then those who took that risk deserve the censure. The reasons or the objectives of taking risks should be clear and easily stated. Risks should be taken to achieve specific goals in the light of possible harms occurring: "We were trying to achieve . . . although, yes, we realised that these harms might occur."

Having goals and objectives for a patient or client is surely a central part of the nursing task. Some might argue that it is enough to justify the risk after the event, if and when it goes wrong. This is unwise. The reasons may show that it was a wise decision and that the same decision would be made again. That could be enough to show that the risk-taking did not cause, in legal terms, the loss suffered. (See the section on causation in the previous chapter on the law of negligence). But it could show enough carelessness to justify disciplinary proceedings. When a court or tribunal assesses the quality of a risk-taking *decision*, it can only consider the information and reasons that were actually available at the time to the decision-maker. Disciplinary action should be concerned with poor decisions whether or not harm results.

The range of benefits and losses

A patient gets his wish to return home quickly. That is a benefit to consider in assessing the risk of early discharge. But it should not be limited to that. There could be benefits to other members of his family. It is not just the patient or client who may benefit or be harmed, but relatives and others. And it is not just the return home itself, but what it may lead to; for example, a reconciled marriage, preserved employment, pets not destroyed, skills maintained, accommodation retained. Risk-taking schemes should consider both the range of people who may be affected and the ways in which they may be affected. It should also consider the 'knock-on' effects. Somebody else may be able to use the vacated bed. Funds may be allocated to another desirable activity.

A duty to risk?

A reason for early discharge, for example, may be pressure on beds. The reason for allowing a client sharp tools may be a belief in the right to take risks or the need to show trust. These are not disreputable reasons. There are pressures on nurses from the government to make best use of scarce resources. There are care philosophies, such as normalisation, suggesting how nurses should behave and patients should be regarded. So, to an extent, nurses are being told or encouraged to take risks. Community care is a policy full of risks, although highly desirable. These duties should be acknowledged in risk-taking schemes and decisions. They are an important dimension affecting behaviour. Indeed, they may demonstrate that it is a dilemma rather than a risk. Judges should consider the duties to act in particular ways.

Sometimes care policies or goals sound empty or vague: "We believe our patients have a right to individuality, respect and a valued environment." But who doesn't? That policy may actually be empty, or there may be a series of documents or models which show what those proud goals mean in actual daily life. The more that these goals and policies can be converted into statements of what people will actually be doing, then the easier it will be to get them accepted as genuine and important duties in the risk assessment.

Manipulating risks

Risks do not exist in a vacuum. They can be manipulated. The risks involved in not asking a doctor to arrange an admission to hospital can be reduced by ensuring that the patient or an informal carer has a relevant telephone number and knows what signs to look for and how to respond. Just as the amount or likelihood of the harms can be reduced, so can the amount and likelihood of the benefits be maximised. Instead of having a vague objective for a patient of living in an ordinary house in the community, *specific* objectives could be cooking, washing and shopping for himself. The more things that could go right, the more justifiable the decision to risk.

It also becomes possible to re-analyse a risk as a dilemma. Moving someone from a large, rundown institution into an unfamiliar community is facing up to a dilemma. Nurses must do something. Staying there is not good enough, something must be done. Government or health authority policies, scarce resources, professional standards – all can make a risk better analysed as a dilemma.

Informed consent

Getting the patient's informed consent is good practice and it helps to show that the decision to risk was wise. The patient stands to gain or lose, and agrees with the decision. Similarly, colleagues' opinions would help to show that it was not just an individual's opinion.

The decision

No help can be given with the final decision. That is for the individual case and the individual nurse. But any decision to risk should be presented as a decision to obtain certain goals, for certain reasons, in the knowledge of the possibility of (and being prepared for) some harms.

Although this strategy does not solve individual cases, it could encourage more risk-taking. It emphasises the importance of accurately representing the risk and the benefits that could come from it. It discourages the overdramatising which may result from concentration on what might go wrong. It can lead to risk decisions being taken proudly rather than with a measure of shame and regret.

But, it may be objected, this long and detailed approach cannot be used every time a nurse has to decide whether a patient can, for example, go to the toilet unaided. Very true: it could often be impractical. It is an aid to decision-making, not a substitute. But, even if not used in detail, it could aid thinking about risks. What are the advantages of letting the patient go unaided? It encourages thought and responsibility. It justifies drawing the line when insufficient potential benefits can be demonstrated. It can help justify judgements when nurses are pressed to take decisions with which they disapprove. And it should encourage self-esteem through nurses realising the number of risk-taking judgements they make.

18

Primary nursing: an individual approach to patient allocation

Andrew Gibbs, RMN
Nurse Teacher, Wycombe Health Authority

When our acute psychiatric ward implemented a system of primary nursing, it replaced a workbook in which tasks to be undertaken that day were listed, along with the names of nurses allocated those tasks. This had been intended to give ward activity a measure of preplanning to allow nurses to organise their day effectively. The system reflected a task-oriented approach to care, focusing on the complexity of the task rather than the patient's needs. Accountability was for task completion, with responsibility for decision-making resting with the ward sister or nurse in charge. It was decided to implement a system of team nursing, which would focus on the patients' total needs.

Team nursing

A team of nurses were given responsibility for the planning and implementation of care for a group of patients. However, problems soon became apparent with the new system. There was constant swapping of patients between teams, in an effort to maintain balanced workloads, and overall responsibility still seemed to rest with the team leader or nurse in charge. Care became fragmented, complex channels of communication were needed and it was unclear who had responsibility for patients.

Dissatisfaction with team nursing in Minnesota (Manthey, 1980) brought about the original development of primary nursing systems, which are advocated as effective organisational frameworks (Castledine, 1982; Lee, 1975; Ellis, 1982; Ashley, 1986; Tutton, 1986). It is particularly seen to enhance the nurse–patient relationship in psychiatry (Ritter, 1987) and said to minimise the institutionalising effects of hospitalisation (Armitage, 1985).

Primary nursing

We decided to implement a primary nursing system which addressed the four elements of responsibility, communication, care giver as care planner and patient allocation (Tutton, 1986). I will concentrate on patient allocation, as the development of such a framework within a traditional hospital service often produces difficulties which seem insurmountable – so much so that the term 'primary nursing' is occasionally used to describe a modified team approach (Green, 1983, Cavill, 1981). The distinction between team and primary nursing is important, as there is evidence to suggest that in some circumstances team nursing may deteriorate into task allocation with its attendant limitations (Manthey, 1980).

Patient allocation problems

Staff organisation and the distribution of responsibilities within a nursing team is an issue raised by the Nursing Process Evaluation Working Group (1987). They see the nature of patient allocation as an important facet of ward organisation, a means by which nurses can make the transition from task-centred work to patient-centred care.

This type of patient-centred approach has been apparent for some time and was developing prior to the widespread introduction of the nursing process. In 1975, Mathews, in an extensive study of patient allocation described benefits for both nurses and patients. Patients felt their relationship with individual nurses had improved, giving them a greater feeling of safety and less anxiety, which in turn gave them more time to rest. Nursing staff felt that their care became more patient-centred rather than ward-centred, which produced more cohesive care delivery. As individual needs became more apparent, procedures such as drug administration became more meaningful, rather then dull routines. This greater involvement produced a feeling of improved systems of information with an appropriate emphasis on management techniques.

Patient allocation and the nursing process are complementary. Many authors have described their versions of patient allocation when implementing individualised care. Generally this has involved sub-dividing patients and staff into small groups (Jones, 1982; Green, 1983; Cavill, 1981). Each group has a team leader who coordinates patient care and supervises standards of care within the group.

The charge nurse or sister takes a supervisory and organisational role directing the workload and monitoring the results. The nurse in charge needs to constantly check and monitor learners' and untrained staff's activities and written work (Wright, 1985), and closely supervise those staff whose allocation to patients demands care skills beyond their experience (Jones, 1982). Another responsibility is to allocate workload to team members (Cavill, 1981). This situation, where the nurse in charge is the focus of communication, control and accountability seemed unsatisfactory within a primary nursing system.

Organisational problems

Further problems we were encountering in the team approach were reflected in nursing articles on the topic. There was a tendency to resort to task allocation when organisational problems arose, such as staff shortages or too few experienced staff on duty (Wright, 1985). It was also difficult to include night staff in the system (Mathews, 1975). The heavily structured format appeared to minimise the scope for self-development of nursing staff, as group needs took priority over individual learning needs. The off-duty was also organised so that one member of each of the teams was on duty each shift. This complex planning led to less overall flexibility within the staff group.

Far from the nursing staff becoming responsible and accountable for their own work, it appeared that our efforts had created a structure which produced such a need for conformity within it that patients' needs could not be met effectively. We had wanted to develop a system of individualised care that emphasised individual nurses' responsibility, decision making capabilities, and desire to consolidate existing skills and develop further through therapeutic relationships with patients. Our difficulties were:

- Centralised responsibility.
- Focus on structure rather than patients' needs.
- Undesirable conformity.
- Lack of recognition of the nurse as an individual.
- Lack of clarity regarding day to day responsibility for care planning.
- Uncertainty about change of role.

Selective allocation

We decided to devise a more satisfactory system. Smaller groups would meet to brainstorm ideas which would be bought to larger group meetings twice weekly. This seemed an effective way of generating new ideas and ensuring all staff were consulted and involved. Finally, we agreed that our system of primary nursing would involve only first level nurses as primary nurses, which seemed to be in accord with rule 18 of Nurses, Midwives and Health Visitors Act (1983).

As staff had differing experience and expertise, we decided that the primary nurses would take responsibility for assessment, care planning and evaluation at all times; be responsible for implementing care while on duty and ensuring effective implementation while off duty. They would do this by providing clearly written care plans which would act as nursing prescriptions in their absence.

Nursing staff would be allocated to patients on two levels – long term and day-to-day. The primary nurses would allocate themselves to patients on their admission to the ward. They would then act as primary nurse throughout that patient's stay on the ward, supported by an associate carer who had also selected the patient. The associate carer could be a first or second level nurse or a nursing auxiliary. The relationship with the primary nurse would be educational with a mutual sharing of ideas and experience, rather than a deputising role in the absence of the primary nurse.

Selecting patients

When selecting patients staff were asked to pay attention to their current workload and that of their colleagues, their relationship with the patient and the potential to apply existing skills or develop new ones. The selection process allowed them to regulate their workload and control their learning needs, while the negotiable aspects of the system encouraged sharing by discussion, with potential to practise skills in assertiveness, compromise and confrontation. There was also scope for staff of differing experiences, status and outlook to work together. This increased the potential for learning through role modelling and stimulated nurse–patient relationships based on interest and self-motivation rather than imposition and direction.

---

1. Each nurse selects a number of patients with whom to act as primary nurse.
2. Each member of staff selects a number of patients with whom to act as carer.

Patient's Name	Primary Nurse	Assoc. Carer
A	Jones	Clarke
B	Smith	Robinson
C	Robinson	Smith
D	Clarke	Jones
E	Jones	Clarke
F	Smith	Robinson

These selections should be made with regard to:
a) Current workload of self.
b) Current workload of others.
c) Dependency of patient.
d) Nurse's relationship with patient.

Figure 1. Patients were allocated a nurse and associate carer.

Selective Allocation.

Day by Day Nursing Interventions.

A chart is compiled as follows:

Patient	1st Jan. am	pm	n	2nd Jan. am	pm	n	3rd Jan. am	pm	n	4th Jan. am	pm	n	
A													H
B													I
C													G H
D													L
E													O
F													W

Nurses select the patients for whom they wish to implement care for that shift. Signing their name next to a patient for a shift indicates an acceptance of overall responsibility for the implementation of care for that shift and to meet any contingencies. They must also communicate significant changes to the primary nurse. In this way there is record of responsibility for all patients at all times.

Primary nurses must always select their own patients when on duty. In the absence of primary nurses, assoc. carers must always select their own patients when on duty.

Figure 2. A chart showed patients' names, dates and shift.

On a day-to-day basis, primary nurses allocated themselves to their own patients. In their absence the associate carer stepped in to implement care for that shift (Figure 1). If neither were on duty, another member of staff allocated themselves to the patient. To clarify the allocations made on any day, a chart was compiled showing patients' names, the date and shifts as shown in Figure 2. Signing their name next to a patient's for a shift indicated acceptance of responsibility for the implementation of care for that shift. The allocation list for each shift, when completed, was displayed where patients could see it. Staff were also expected to introduce themselves to their allocated patients at the beginning of each shift to generate a plan of action. Any change considered significant was reported to the primary nurse via daily progress notes, with the onus resting with the primary nurse to seek further information relevant to the patients' future care.

Supervision and management

On each shift a registered nurse acted as a coordinator, enabling the daily activity to run smoothly, dealing with general enquiries (or directing them to the relevant primary nurse), offering support to staff either by discussing specific incidents or giving practical help such as assistance with lifting and the administration of medication.

In this way a record was kept of responsibility and accountability throughout the patient's stay in hospital. The system's flexibility made it operable over a 24 hour period regardless of the number of staff on duty. Staff also retained their individuality and the right to request an off-duty pattern which suited their needs.

The nurse in charge of the ward was free from organisational activities such as directing and regulating workloads. The off-duty rota was easier and could be delegated to others and the initiative for decision making and learning was with individual staff, which allowed the nurse in charge more time to act as a clinical resource who could monitor and supervise standards of practice. Monitoring the selective allocation system allowed the nurse in charge to review patterns of allocation, highlighting areas of expertise or avoidance. This information was helpful in identifying relevant teaching input.

Selective allocation explicitly states individual responsibility, allowing nurses to practise and continually develop new skills. Their learning and workload were now shared in a planned way and both were able to link even in times of staff shortage.

Evaluating the system

The system was evaluated in an informal, subjective way, which, while it may be a disadvantage, was welcomed by both staff and patients. Doctors said they found it mildly annoying that they had to seek out different nurses to discuss different patients, and that this could be time consuming. However, the system seemed to enable proactive rather than reactive care planning, and appeared particularly useful in the care of quiet, withdrawn patients who receive only minimal care under traditional systems (Altschul, 1978). Patients who are often labelled 'demanding' found it helpful to have a designated nurse to approach who was more likely to deal with the factors motivating the demanding behaviour rather than treat the patient as unpopular (Stockwell, 1976). Overall, it was easier for the nurse in charge to identify 'unpopular' patients and discuss the staff dynamics that may contribute to their demanding behaviour. Patients also soon identified 'their' nurse.

Despite these positive comments, the system had many problems. The night staff refused to become involved, for reasons which are unclear, and competition to take on more work became, at times, quite destructive. Some nurses felt that others were 'not pulling their weight'.

Staff shortage

An acute staff shortage highlighted the fact that when staff were brought in from another ward or an agency, the system enabled them to play an effective part in giving care. However, the shortage led to a deterioration in long term allocation and reduced flexibility in off-duty planning. When the senior nurse left, the system collapsed completely, but 18 months later, a slightly modified selective allocation system has been re-introduced.

I feel the positive aspects of the system outweigh the negative and that more effective management of change may have enhanced the possibilities of the system's success. The two essential components of the system are: flexible management who can cope with devolved responsibility, and a balanced skill mix. If these are present, I believe the system may enhance delivery of care in any environment.

References

Altschul, A. (1972) *Patient Nurse Interaction.* Churchill Livingstone, Edinburgh.
Armitage, P. (1985) Primary care. *Nursing Times* **81,** 38, 36-7.
Ashley, J. (1985) From team nursing to individual care. *Nursing Mirror,* **160,** 18, 20-21.
Casledene, G. (1985) Defending the all rounder. *Nursing Times,* **81,** 84.
Cavill, C. and Johnson N. (1977) Steps towards the process. *Nursing Times,* 2091.
DHSS (1987) Report of the nursing process evaluation working group. HMSO, London.
Ellis, E. (1982) The nurse's accountability. *Nursing Times,* **154,** 21, 33-35.
Green, B. (1983) Primary nursing in psychiatry. *Nursing Times,* **79,** 3, 25.
Jones, J. (1982) The nursing process in psychiatry. *Nursing Times,* **78,** 30, 1273-75.
Lee, M. (1979) Towards better care. *Nursing Times,* **75,** 51, 133-6.
Manthey, M. (1980) A theoretical framework for primary nursing. *Journal of Nursing Administration,* **10,** 6, 11-15.
Mathews, A. (1975) Patient allocation. *Nursing Times,* **71,** 29, 65-8.
Ritter, S. (1987) Primary nursing in mental illness. *Nursing Mirror,* **160,** 17, 20-21.
Stockwill, F. (1976) The Unpopular Patient. RCN, London.
Tutton, L. (1986) What is primary nursing? *the Professional Nurse,* **2,** 39-41.
Wright, S. (1985) Special assignment. *Nursing Times,* **81,** 36-7.

19

The role of the associate nurse

Sarah Burns, RGN
Lecturer/Practitioner, John Radcliffe Hospital, Oxford

Since primary nursing was implemented at the John Radcliffe Hospital, much attention has been focused on the primary nurse role (Tutton, 1986; MacMahon 1987). Primary nursing is the system whereby all patients and clients are allocated to a primary nurse on entering care. This nurse is then responsible for their nursing round-the-clock as long as it is needed. She is both responsible and accountable for the care she plans and gives. However, the primary nurse can rarely be the sole provider of this care and is therefore assisted by associate nurses. It is important to examine the role of the associate nurse, as without a clear understanding, it may be interpreted as having low status, which we at the John Radcliffe have found not to be true.

Throughout the period of nursing development those nurses who function exclusively as associate nurses have coped extremely well with the perceived threat to their own role, which was caused by uncertainty and inexperience making it difficult to see the eventual role clearly. Now we can review some of the changes to our fundamental thinking.

Who should be an associate nurse?
Experience of the associate nurse role is almost a prerequisite to becoming a primary nurse. The potential for personal and professional development is great and, I feel, vital in preparing a primary nurse.

Most of our associate nurses are newly registered or part-time qualified nurses, but student nurses may fill this role as long as they have appropriate supervision. It should also be remembered that the associate nurse may be another primary nurse in the team who is providing cover during a colleague's absence.

Hierarchy
The hierarchical structures which supported our traditional nursing practice have had to be dismantled where they were found to be inhibiting us. For example, our communication network previously meant that the associate nurses discussed nursing care issues with the sister or nurse in charge, who would then decide whether to take the issue to the nurse specialist, doctor or other professional. This inhibited

the development of the associate nurses' confidence and creativity. To combat this all had to work hard to promote and support direct communication, so the associate nurses can initiate discussion with any professionals. We have found the role of sister has become one of advisor on clinical issues rather than major decision-maker.

We have tried to transfer the values and beliefs about the relationship with clients to our relationships with each other. These hinge on the nature of the relationship between the nurse and client – it must be a close partnership, with each party able to identify the other – the notion of 'my nurse' or 'my patient' as Manthey (1970) puts it.

The freedom and comfort required to develop the partnership can be inhibited by an hierarchical nursing team, but an open atmosphere of mutual trust and respect helps partnerships to flourish. It is important to recognise, however, that this is not the whole answer – individual nurses must want to develop these relationships. For many nurses this is uncharted territory and can be perceived as very threatening.

Part of the willingness to participate comes from each member feeling valued as part of the team, a feeling which is very much influenced by the ward sister. Manthey (1970) suggests that the ability of the ward sister to change her role and allow open and free staff relationships to develop is crucial to the overall implementation of a primary nursing system. Regular ward meetings, sometimes with the ward sister disclosing her own fears, worries and triumphs encourage an atmosphere in which other nurses feel able to disclose and share feelings. This open interest in and care of each other is new for many nurses. It is important that all members of the team work to develop an atmosphere in which individuals feel comfortable disclosing their feelings without fear of ridicule or retribution.

Smaller teams

One way of promoting this working relationship is to break the large nursing team into smaller teams. Headed by one or more primary nurses, the rest of the small team is composed of associate nurses. These teams look after a small group of patients within the ward or department, allowing all staff continuity of care – that is looking after the same patients each time they are on duty. Without a team approach, an associate nurse who acts exclusively in that role can find herself looking after one primary nurse's patients one day and another's the next, so she herself does not experience continuity of care.

One associate nurse described this as feeling like a foster mother. Having worked hard at developing a good relationship with one group of clients she had to hand them back to the primary nurse feeling very much as a foster mother might feel when returning a child to its natural mother. Using a team approach means the associate nurse looks after the same group of patients whenever she is on duty.

The diagrams illustrate examples of team membership. In Figure 1, meeting clients' nursing care needs is the responsibility of the primary nurse. The associate nurses assist in carrying out this care, especially when the primary nurse is off duty. Clarification of care can be elicited from the care plan, but as the associate nurses can have as much continuous contact with the clients as the primary nurse, communication is generally easier, more effective and less open to error or breakdown. Figure 2 illustrates that where there is more than one primary nurse in a team each will 'associate' for the other when she or he is off duty, thus acting in both roles on one shift. The associate nurse will 'associate' for both primary nurses in their joint absence.

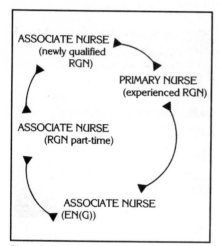

Figure 1. The primary nurse is responsible for nursing care in this team, helped by the associate nurses.

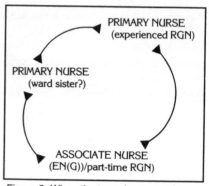

Figure 2. When the team has more than one primary nurse, they will 'associate' for each other, both helped by the associate nurse.

The feeling of belonging gained from the team approach, of contributing to the care of a group of clients, of receiving acknowledgement of one's endeavours all reflect Maslow's hierarchy of needs. The stage is then set for the creative contributions of the associate nurse in giving highly personalised nursing care.

Guidelines

For individual nurses to reach this point, some guidelines are necessary. Up-to-date job descriptions and standards help clarify what is and what is not expected, but it is important that individual nurses feel that acknowledgement is made of past experience and special abilities. Setting personal targets from job performance reviews is helpful in this area, which is ripe for development by ward sisters.

Associate nurses are essential members of the nursing team within a primary nursing system. They are accountable for their own practices, and their contribution to clients' care is active rather than passive. They are trained to use professional judgement in their clients' interests, and to evaluate their own practice. The level of decision-making expected from associate nurses can vary, but all team members should be clear about it. They, and nurse managers, must also acknowledge that some associate nurses may have extensive experience and expertise.

If the associate nurse role is to emerge as a positive and valued role within a primary nursing system, all members of the team need to examine all aspects of their behaviour which might inhibit freedom of speech and action in other team members. Otherwise the associate nurse will merely be the primary nurses' handmaiden.

References
Manthey, M. (1970) A return to the concept of my nurse and my patient. *Nursing Forum*, **9**, 1, 65-83.
Manthey, M. (1980) *The Practice of Primary Nursing*. Blackwell Scientific, New York.
Maslow, A. (1970) *Motivation and Personality* (2nd Ed.) Harper Row, New York.

20

What are the legal implications of extended nursing roles?

Susannah Derrick, RGN
Senior Staff Nurse, Intensive Care Unit, St Mary's Hospital, London

Recent advances in medical technology have led to constant demands being made on both the knowledge and skills of nurses. This is highlighted in 'high tech' areas of nursing such as intensive care and renal units.

Nurses have a complex role in these areas. It requires not only competence in providing basic care, support and education to patient and family, but also a high level of theoretical knowledge and practical skill to understand and contribute to treatment. The role of the specialist nurse encompasses many procedures which have previously been considered within the medical domain, such as venepuncture and emergency defibrillation.

The legal issues

I would suggest that nurses working in these areas extend their role willingly. However, although they are trained for practice, they may not fully appreciate the legal issues surrounding it.

A research case study carried out using RGNs in an intensive/cardiac care unit as a sample population supports this suggestion and has provided factual information on the degree of knowledge and appreciation of the legal implications of the extended role held by this specific population (Derrick, 1987). The study also presents a reasonable overview of the RGN population as a whole, as it demonstrated the broad background and wide range of hospitals and health authorities in which the sample had previously worked.

What is an extended role?

An extended role can be described as one which is not included in basic training. They have developed for various reasons; the most obvious is development of new technology and treatment. However, economic factors can not be overlooked – nursing manpower may be cheaper than medical.

In the light of the change and extension of the nursing role the DHSS, medical and nursing professional organisations attempted to clarify the situation. The DHSS issued a circular in 1977 explaining the legal implications and training requirements (DHSS, 1977), and this was supported by a publication from the RCN and BMA (1978). These documents set out some clear guidelines for the management of extended roles for nurses, and are summarised by Rowden (1987.)

The guidelines stress the need for joint discussions, mutual trust and respect between professions and state that extension of role must be in the interests of patient care. An opinion often aired is that on a busy ward where staffing levels are low, skilled nurses should not be using precious time administering intravenous drugs.

The circular also states that 'Work which has hitherto been carried out by doctors ought therefore to be delegated to nurses only when:-
a) The nurse has been specifically and adequately trained for the performance of the new task and she agrees to undertake it;
b) this training has been recognised as satisfactory by the employing Authority;
c) the new task has been recognised by the professions and by the employing Authority as a task which may be properly delegated to a nurse;
d) the delegating doctor has been assured of the competence of the individual nurse concerned.'

It also states:- 'In order to be successful and safe such delegation should be in the context of a clearly defined policy . . . and it should be made known in writing to all staff who are likely to be involved.

These points should be considered very carefully and with particular reference to the Department of Health document, the Ministerial Group on Junior Doctors' hours (Department of Health, 1990). Reduction in the hours worked by junior doctors is a subject which rightly gains a great deal of support, and this document presents recommendations to achieve this. However, it is interesting to note one such recommendation in the document. II. Recommendations for Action No. 6 "the UK Health Departments should issue guidelines to health authorities and boards as follows" (d) "in consultation with the UKCC for Nursing, Midwifery and Health Visiting and the Royal Colleges of Nursing and Midwifery, on the need for reviews of local policies concerning activities which appropriately qualified nurses and midwives may reasonably undertake further to improve the quality of patient care. Where such local policies do not exist, arrangements should be made for them to be instituted."

Could this imply transfer of 'activities' or practices from a medical to a nursing responsibility?

It is important that nursing management and individual nurses are flexible to change and are able to respond to the needs of their patients in the light of increasing knowledge and advancing technology. But it is essential they understand the implications of the changes in practice.

Certification

A certificate of competence is issued for some extended role procedures. Unlike the administration of intravenous drugs (Breckenbridge, 1976) many procedures do not require certification in some authorities but do in others. Certification is not a legal requirement, but it does serve a worthwhile purpose.

Each individual nurse has a choice whether or not to extend her or his role. It can be generally accepted that any nurse choosing to work in specialised fields expects, and is willing to undertake an extended role, and with adequate training should be fully aware of the medical and nursing implications of her or his actions. Comment is rarely made, however, about the importance and need for training to enable nurses to appreciate the legal implications of their actions.

Law and the nurse

Accountability   "Each registered nurse, midwife and health visitor is accountable for his or her practice" (UKCC, 1984). Accountability means being answerable for work, decisions about work and being professionally responsible for the standard of practice. Nurses are first and foremost legally responsible for each and every nursing action undertaken or omitted, and must practise in accordance with the same standard of care of a reasonably prudent nurse practising under the same or similar circumstances. *Primary liability* is held by the individual nurse for her or his own actions.

It is possible for nurses to be persuaded or pressurised into carrying out treatment or procedures – extending their role – either to be helpful, to save time or 'to keep the peace', particularly when wards are busy or staffing levels are low. In such instances both medical and nursing staff should have the consequences of the unauthorised practise brought to their attention. Protecting one another from primary liability is a duty everyone should adopt, and be thanked for, albeit as an afterthought.

Greater awareness of legal issues surrounding nursing and the extension of the nursing role has developed in recent years. The number of study days and articles published on this subject has undoubtedly increased the level of interest and understanding.

In March 1989 the UKCC for for Nursing, Midwifery and Health Visiting published an Advisory Document 'Exercising Accountability'. It is designed to offer a framework to assist nurses, midwives and health visitors to consider ethical aspects of professional practise and is available free to all on the UKCC's professional register (UKCC, 1989).

Negligence   Negligence is divided into three main components (Rea, 1987):

● **The duty of care** The legal duty of care encompasses the professional, moral, ethical and sociological duties of care within which nursing operates. It is what the nurse is required to do under the terms of her

contract of employment. Deviation from this in any way is negligence.
- **The breach of the duty** This is the alleged wrongdoing.
- **The resultant damage** The damage to the patient must be the result of the breach of the duty of care.

The law relating to negligence principally seeks to identify conduct which does not reach an acceptable professional standard. If injury results from such conduct the possibility of an action for damages (compensation) arises. Liability to pay damages may be shouldered by the individual, covered by an insurance company or by membership of a professional organisation which offers legal liability insurance to its members.

Vicarious liability

In the DHSS circular (1977), and in law, it is made clear that any role extension *must* be approved officially by the employing authority. In the United Kingdom (Master-Servant Statutes) "the law takes the view that the master will accept responsibility for the actions of servants, where the servant is working in accordance with the policies agreed by master and servant" (Rowden, 1987). Within the NHS the employing authority is the master and the nurse the servant. It is normally accepted that the senior nurse will act on behalf of the authority.

The health authority will accept responsibility for the actions of nurses when they are working within policies agreed by both parties. It is suggested therefore that it may be good practice for nurses to be certificated for extended role procedures. In the extended role, a certificate not only facilitates education and the maintenance of a high standard of care but is proof of competence and of the authority's knowledge and agreement for the nurse to practise.

If the authority/employer is to accept legal liability for the action of the nurse/employee, it is necessary that the authority should know exactly the role being practised and agree to it. This is known as *vicarious liability* (sometimes called secondary liability). It is essential to confirm in writing any extension of role. It is too easy for confusion to arise where verbal agreements are concerned. How many times has a doctor been heard to say 'I will cover you'? Doctors are *not* permitted by their defence organisations to take responsibility for the actions of nurses. Documenting the extent and boundaries of an extended role may seem tedious and bureaucratic, but it is in the interests of practitioners and patients alike.

Ensuring knowledge

It is essential to ensure nurses have an appreciation and thorough understanding of the implications of the extension of the nursing role. With the ever increasing expectation that all nurses at all levels extend their role further, I would make the following recommendations:

- Individuals and management must be alerted to the need for more education.

- The teaching of the legal aspects of nursing should be incorporated into basic training and all nurses should be encouraged to question their own knowledge and safeguard their own practise.

- Incorporation of the legal implications in the criteria of certification for an extended role procedure would ensure awareness of the policy and requirements of the issuing health authority/employer.

- Attempts should be made to find time and finance to increase the number of study days, teaching sessions, workshops and discussions available.

Each registered nurse, midwife and health visitor is accountable for his or her practice. It is every nurse's individual responsibility to understand the legal implications underlying that accountability. Do you?

References

Department of Health (1990) *Heads of Agreement. Ministerial Group on Junior Doctor's Hours.* December. DoH, London.

Derrick, S.M. (1987) Unpublished case study on nurses' appreciation of the legal implications of taking an extended role.

DHSS (1977) *The extending role of the clinical nurse – legal implications and training requirements.* DHSS, London.

RCN/BMA (1978) *The Duties and Position of the Nurse.* RCN, London.

Rea, K. (1987) Negligence. *Nursing*, **3**, 576.

UKCC (1984) *Code of Professional Conduct for the Nurse, Midwife and Health Visitor.* UKCC, London.

UKCC (1989) *Exercising Accountability.* UKCC, London.

Quality Assurance

21

Quality of nursing care: meaning and measures

Nancy Dixon, BSc, MA, CPQA
Consultant in Quality Healthcare, Romsey

Nurses have made major efforts to develop standards and to audit quality of nursing care over several years. Now, NHS policymakers and managers, as well as the professions, are joining together to make quality a cornerstone of the NHS reforms. Amidst the frenzied activities generated by various national and local initiatives on standards and audit, which were launched in the context of the reforms, a clear meaning of the concept of quality, as it applies to health care, has not yet emerged. In the absence of clarity about the concept, it is possible that confusion also may emerge about the most useful means to achieve quality.

The meaning of quality

A number of prominent authors have reviewed the meaning of quality in health care and have offered their views. In a review of meanings of quality in health care, Reerink stated that defining quality is a mission impossible (Reerink, 1990). Quality is like beauty or colour, an intangible to which each individual ascribes meaning based on personal values, beliefs, and experiences.

The first remote references to the concept of quality in health care in modern history were by Florence Nightingale, and others of her time, who argued for the collection of statistics about the sick in order to draw possible conclusions about the results of health care (Nightingale, 1863). This suggestion of the value of outcomes, in relation to judgements about quality of health care was taken up and developed by an American surgeon, E A Codman, who exhorted his colleagues to study the outcomes of their surgical procedures a year following the operations (Codman, 1914).

More recently, thinkers about quality of health care have developed broader concepts of the meaning of quality, no doubt reflecting the complexity of major health care systems and technologies. For example, Donabedian (1987) whose work is recognised internationally, distinguished between quality of health care for individuals and that for entire communities. Care of individual patients is judged primarily on the degree to which practitioners provide treatment capable of producing the greatest improvement that science can achieve. For communities, Donabedian widens the attributes of quality to include access to care and equitable distribution of care.

Caper (1988) identified three components of quality:

1. Efficacy, ie, whether or not a particular intervention accomplishes the goal for its use.
2. Appropriateness, ie, whether a particular intervention is used only when its cost can be balanced by its benefit for an individual patient.
3. Interpersonal, supportive, and psychological aspects of the provider-patient relationship.

In a prominent medical lecture about quality, Bowen expressed a view that quality should include an "enduring concern for patients as people", however, he acknowledged that a desire to extend the healing touch must be tempered by the limits of society's resources (Bowen, 1987).

The results of a major research study on quality assurance in the USA, which was carried out by the Institute of Medicine, have recently been published. As a basis for the study, the researchers devised an operational definition of quality of care which is the degree to which health services for individuals and populations increase the likelihood of desired health outcomes and are consistent with current professional knowledge. (Lohr and Schroedes, 1990).

These various definitions present a few major themes about quality of health care. These themes are as follows:

- Practitioners tend to focus on individual patients, whereas those with accountability to the public as a whole tend to focus on communities of people with health care needs.
- Resource limitations require compromise between individuals and communities, in regard to meeting health care needs.
- Resource limitations dictate that one component of quality is the appropriateness of interventions provided to individual patients.
- Quality must be judged at least by outcome, ie, "the greatest improvement that science can achieve".
- The perception of quality by the recipient of a health care service, particularly in relation to the recipient's expectations, is a component of quality.

In conclusion, quality is concerned with individuals as well as with groups. Quality implies a focus on outcomes and opinion from recipients of services. Also, resource constraints may have led thinkers to suggest that quality also may imply the least amount of intervention needed to achieve a desired outcome.

Implications for nursing standards and audit

Donabedian (1982) wrote about "the bridge that connects the grand abstractions (of quality) . . . with the actual business of passing a judgement on the quality of care in any particular instance". He labelled the bridge the "criteria and standards to be used for assessing quality". Thus, agreeing on practical statements of what quality means becomes the key to measuring quality of health care.

For some nursing quality assurance practitioners, measures of quality are synonymous with standards of quality (Whelan, 1991). Standards of care are valid, acceptable definitions of the quality of nursing care, ie, statements of what good nursing care should be (Sale, 1990). Commonly accepted models for the development of standards require that a standard statement consist of structure, process, and outcome criteria to be used to judge achievement of the standard (Kendall and Kitson, 1986; Mason, 1984; Sale, 1990). The assessment of actual practice, using standards of care, is the audit process.

However, the selection of specific measures of quality as well as the selection of the method for audit depend upon which guiding concept of quality professionals choose to adopt. For example, using the Institute of Medicine (IOM) definition earlier cited (Lohr and Schroeder, 1990), the implications for nursing standards and nursing audit are shown in Table 1.

Idea about quality	Implication for audit process
Degree to which health services	Requires **measurement** to a relatively **precise.**
for **individuals and populations**	Enables **both indepth** study of individuals **and surveillance** of group.
increase the likelihood	Considers **efficacy** and **appropriateness** of interventions.
of **desired**	Includes **patient/public** input on **expectations.**
health outcomes	Focuses on **results to patients,** not practitioner tasks.
and are **consistent with current knowledge**	Reflects up-to-date practices.

Table 1. Implications for nursing standards and audit.

Commitment to this illustrative concept of quality of health care requires a more demanding approach to audit than other concepts of quality might require. The IOM definition of quality for example, might obligate nurses to seek patients' views and/or public views on their 'desired' outcomes. It places significantly more emphasis on outcomes of care than on structure or process considerations. Most critically for nurses, the definition introduces a discipline of evaluating the efficacy and appropriateness of specific aspects of care. For a nursing audit process the definition means that nurses will need to ask 'Are we doing the *right* things?' as well as 'Are we doing the *same* things?'.

Contrasting philosophies of audit

Doctors and health care professionals are beginning to consider how various theories of quality assurance or quality management apply to health care.

One theory of achieving quality requires systematic assessment of all key aspects of performance against comprehensive standards, ie, 'quality by inspection'. The measurement process may be internally or externally conducted. But its purpose is to define virtually all aspects, ie, structure, processes, *and* outcomes of performance through standards, and then to assess performance against all the standards. The result of this approach to measuring quality is a 'score card' of performance, which is sometimes designed to enable comparisons among units subjected to the same inspection. Performance which does not meet standards or varies widely from the norm is thought to represent a 'problem' which must be resolved.

An alternative theory starts with a different premise, ie, that quality is a moving target which can nearly always be improved. Quality is not measured by conformance to fixed comprehensive standards which define quality. Standards may exist and be available as reference points. Rather, in the alternative theory, quality is expressed by indicators of performance which are invented solely for audit purposes to judge whether or not quality is improving. Whereas the first theory tends to be aimed at exposing bad practice, the second tends to be aimed at continuously improving existing levels of quality (Berwick, 1989; Smith, 1990).

Consider how these theories might apply to nursing audit. For example, in many approaches to nursing audit, an assumption is made that the purpose of the quality assessment is to evaluate the implementation of all nursing standards. However, this assumption is wasteful of the most precious resource nurses have in regard to quality assessment: their time. Is it valid to assume that all nursing standards are of equal importance and should be equally weighted as bases for nursing quality assessment? In truth, a few nursing standards are of absolutely vital importance in terms of their known effects on the achievement of desired health outcomes of patients. Many nursing standards are of moderate importance, and for some, there may be little scientific evidence that conformance with the standard actually has any effect on patients' outcomes.

In summary, the discipline of selecting a guiding concept of the meaning of quality and a guiding philosophy of audit may affect not only the process of audit but its ultimate value to patient care.

Standards versus indicators as a basis for nursing audit

Standards of care, as already referred to, are one means of defining quality of nursing care (Sale, 1990). They specify what patient care should be provided, how care should be provided, and how achievement of the results of that care, ie, outcomes, can be judged. Nursing standards rely heavily on clinical knowledge and judgement.

Audit indicators, on the other hand, specify what and how patient care should be audited. They express nurses' expectations of quality of patient care for audit purposes only. Audit indicators rely on the objectives for particular audits and on the strategies to be used to collect data related to the indicator. Indicators act as 'screens' or 'flags' through which quality of patient care can be evaluated. They are used to identify cases, situations, or circumstances about which staff wish to know the exact level of quality being provided. An audit indicator implies that a standard of care exists but it may not measure compliance with the entire standard (Dixon, 1991).

To be useful for audit, an indicator should be consistent with the following characteristics:

- It should be clinically valid, that is, based on current clinical knowledge, clinical judgement, and clinical experience.
- It should be sufficiently specific and well-defined that it contains no ambiguity in meaning.
- It should be objective, to the degree possible.
- It should be relevant and applicable to the group of patients covered by the audit.
- It should enable efficient data collection (Fromberg, 1988).

Constructing

An audit indicator is constructed using four components as follows:

- The specific **aspect** of care or service being audited, described with the minimum essential or most important evidence that would satisfy nurses that the quality of nursing care being provided is appropriate. Aspects of care or service can be nursing processes, or outcomes, or, when appropriate, structural or resource requirements.
- A **percentage** which states, *in advance*, the degree of compliance desired or expected, for audit purposes, for the aspect of nursing care or service being audited. The percentage can be a target percentage which nurses are aiming for: an acceptable percentage as cited in the literature, or 100% or 0% used arbitrarily for the critical aspects of care which should pertain to *all* patients *all* of the time or to *no* patients *none* of the time.
- Any **exceptions** which are common clinically acceptable reasons or circumstances that would account for a failure to conform with the aspect of nursing care or service.
- Definitions of terms used to judge conformance with the aspect of care or exception, including synonyms or numerical values, and instructions for data sources to be used in the audit.

An example of a subject for an audit indicator might be hospital acquired infection. The presence of infection is the aspect of care being measured. If the nursing staff sets a target that no more than five per cent of patients should develop an infection in hospital, the audit indicator's percentage would be 5%. If the staff researched the literature and found that an average of nine per cent of patients develop infection in hospital, they might choose 9% as the indicator percentage. Or if nurses were interested in doing everything possible to reduce hospital acquired infection, they may wish to review every single incidence of such infection to determine if any could have been prevented. In this approach, the indicator percentage would be 0%, for audit purposes only. Nurses would have to agree on the signs and symptoms they would accept as evidence of infection and the time frame in which the symptoms could occur and be thought of as hospital acquired. They also would have to agree on where evidence of infection will be documented reliably.

Choosing measures of quality for audit indicators

If nursing staff wish to adopt a nursing audit philosophy which is flexible and does not require monitoring of total compliance with all standards, nurses may need to think about how to choose measures of nursing quality. One way to make such choices is to think about those aspects of nursing care that are known or believed to have an impact on the overall quality of patient care. There are several ways through which impact can be considered. The most common methods are to consider answers to the following question:

- In the specific care setting, what aspects of care are nurses concerned with most frequently? Whether the aspect is a nursing intervention, a nursing outcome, or a nursing resource, if the aspect occurs frequently, there are two immediate implications for audit purposes. First, if an aspect of nursing care is carried out with high frequency, probably a large number of patients are involved. Nurses may wish to use audit to ensure that at least for those large groups of patients, nursing care meets the nurses' and the patients' expectations. Second, a high frequency aspect of care may produce error. Nurses may wish to know precisely their 'error rates' for such aspects of care.
- In the specific care setting, what aspects of nursing care are most associated with risk? Risk means simply that a patient may suffer harm or less than optimal outcome or a decrease in level of functioning in the absence of appropriate care, either by the wrong care being given or by no care being given when it should have been.

There are two ways to consider risk potential for nursing care. First, are there particular individual patients who are at greater risk, from a nursing viewpoint, than others? If so, the audit process should concentrate on these individuals or groups, to ensure that nursing care does not contribute to an even greater risk level. Second, are there some nursing interventions or outcomes which, if not done or achieved properly or if not done or achieved at all, could pose a risk to patients? If so, the audit process should concentrate on those particular aspects of nursing care.

● In the specific care setting, are there any aspects of nursing care which have been related to a problem in the past? A problem in this context could be a serious complaint or a major issue raised by patients, relatives, staff, or management. If there is any lingering doubt as to whether or not the problem or concern is resolved completely, the involved aspects of nursing care are appropriate priorities for the audit process.

Other questions about impact of nursing care can be asked. However, the three described about frequency, risk potential, and patient/staff problems are likely to elicit high priorities for nursing audit. The questions also relate to the IOM definition of quality illustrated earlier. The question are highly likely to require consideration among nurses about aspects of care provided to individual patients versus groups of patients; efficacy and appropriateness of nursing care; patient/public views; patient outcomes; and currency of practice issues.

Developing a vision of quality

Quality is a personal concept defined somewhat differently by each individual. Like beauty, the presence of quality is sometimes what is 'in the eye of the beholder'.

Quality in health care services is no exception to this observation. It is an extremely emotive subject in the context of the NHS. People working in the NHS uniformly support the idea of improving the quality of NHS services provided to the public. However, their perceptions and emotions about quality in the NHS vary considerably, often as guises for their personal political views. For some, quality in the NHS is primarily about timely equity of access to unlimited and free health care by all members of the public. For others, quality is about recapturing the staffing levels which are perceived as being available before the pressure began to increase throughput and reduce costs. For still others, quality is encompassed by following professional standards whether they are implicit or explicit.

Well- intentioned nurses who accept that the day-to-day performance of nursing staff no doubt could be improved often are faced with the pressures of their jobs, the cynicism of co-workers, or the preoccupation of their managers with other matters. In the absence of a clear vision or guiding concept of quality for nursing care and an appropriate approach to measuring the quality of nursing care, nurses' individual efforts to improve quality may be jeopardised. These potential circumstances suggest that nurses need to assume leadership in developing a vision of quality and in measuring day-to-day nursing care in relation to that vision. The use of audit indicators as a basis for striving for continuous improvement of quality should facilitate the process.

References

Berwick, D.M. (1989) Continuous improvement as an ideal in health care. *New English Journal of Medicine*, **320**, 53–6.

Bowen O.R. (1987) What is quality care? *New English Journal of Medicine*, **316**, 1578–80.

Caper, P. (1988) Defining quality in medical care. *Health Affairs*, 7, (1) 49–61.

Codman E.A. (1984) The product of a hospital. *Surgery, Gynaecology and Obstetrics*, **85**, 491–6.

Dixon, N. (1991) *Nursing Audit Primer*. Healthcare Quality Quest, Romsey.

Donabedian, A. (1982) *The Criteria and Standards of Quality. Explorations in Quality Assessment and Monitoring.* Vol II. Ann Arbor: Health Administration Press, 3–6.

Donabedian, A. (1987) Five essential questions frame the management of quality in health care. *Health Management Quality*, **9** (1) 6–9.

Fromberg, R. (1988) *The Joint Commission Guide to Quality Assurance.* Joint Commission on Accreditation of Healthcare Organisations, Chicago.

Kendall, H. and Kitson, A. (1986) Rest assured. *Nursing Times*, **82**, 28–31.

Lohr K.N. and Schroeder S.A. (1990) A strategy for quality assurance in Medicare. *New English Journal of Medicine*, **322**, 707–12.

Mason, E.J. (1984) *How to Write Meaningful Nursing Standards, 2nd Ed.* John Wiley and Sons, New York.

Nightingale, F. (1863) *Notes on Hospitals*, 3rd Ed. Longman, Green, Longman, Roberts, and Green, London.

Reerink, E. (1990) Defining quality of care: mission impossible? *Quality Assurance in Health Care*, **2**, 197–202.

Sale, D. (1990) *Quality Assurance*. Macmillan, Basingstoke.

Smith, R. (1990) Medicine's need for kaizen. Putting quality first. *British Medical Journal*, **301**, 679–80.

Whelan, J. (1991) Troublespots in quality assurance. *Nursing Standard*, **5**, 36–8.

22

What is quality assurance?

Nan Kemp, SRN, RCNT, DIP.N(Lond)
Freelance Consultant, Quality Assurance

Nurses need to set standards of care for their own practice and to be involved in the selection of quality monitoring methodologies. Otherwise others will do this for them. Today many nurses are involved in quality assurance issues. However, with the changes being brought about by the NHS and Community Care Act 1990 and the further emphasis on the work force, nurses must not let themselves become victims of cost containment. Nurses must see it as a challenge to further their practice, whilst ensuring that consideration of cost is just one part of their standard setting strategy (Kemp and Richardson, 1990). An advantage of the new Directories should be the development of a multidisciplinary quality monitoring methodology. This may not be easy, but it could be one of the good things to come out of the changes occurring in the NHS. At times of such change it is important that health professionals adhere to their professional ethics, with all that involves, to ensure that no harm comes to patients, colleagues and the society which they serve.

The importance of evaluating care

With the advent of the new management structure of the National Health Service, there is as never before a need for nurses to question their practice, seek advice and use research findings that will enable them to plan and implement some method of systematically evaluating the care and support given to patients and staff. For, as we enter this new health-care environment, we need to be able to speak with credibility and authority about nursing and to maintain our professional identity. I make no apology for stressing the point that we need to back up what we say with facts, particularly when requesting the use of scarce resources.

In the field of quality assurance, which means to assure the client of quality, there could be an exciting time ahead of us. However, if we do not question what we are doing and why, and develop and/or use tools to measure and enhance our practice, we will "miss the boat" and others may try to do this for us.

Each of us has a responsibility to ensure appropriate standards of patient care, whether we are clinical nurses, managers, or teachers. But how do we know if we are giving quality nursing care? Is it a hunch? Is it what the patient, his family, and others tell us? Is it the result of complaints, accidents, reports, waiting lists, and/or bed occupancy figures, or bequests and letters of appreciation? Is it the sickness/absence or retention of staff?

Setting the standards for care

The answers to these questions are indicators of quality, but do they provide a measurement of care? It can be thought that wards receiving few letters of complaint and many letters of appreciation and where staff are relatively easy to recruit and remain in post for a long time, are those where the quality of nursing care is good. But that is not necessarily the case; it may be, for example, that those wards particularly suit the needs of the staff. The very complexity of patient care, and nursing in particular, makes quality difficult to measure. The quality of nursing care cannot be measured in isolation from the activities of other disciplines; it is only one aspect of patient care and while we may begin to determine the quality of nursing care, that will only give one aspect of the measurement of quality of patient care

We should now be taking it upon ourselves to determine how the nursing component of patient care ought to be measured. It is our responsibility to set our own standards and to develop, or select for use already established, tools for measuring quality; if we do not set the standards, false assumptions may be made by others about the work of nurses.

Measuring the quality of care

How does one set about measuring the quality of care? Donabedian (1966) asked this question of medicine, and his work is central to much of what has since followed in evaluating care. He argued that three major interlocking components affected care, and he called these structure, process, and outcome (Table 1).

- Structure refers to factors within the organisation such as the environment, equipment, staff, and management styles.
- Process is the actual care that the patient/or client receives from the health care team. Process can be measured by the use of patient and nurse interviews, observation of the nursing care, and the examination of Nursing Care records.
- Outcome is the end result of care, the effect on the patient or his family. This is particularly difficult to measure since it relies on the making of some assessment of patient satisfaction and understanding. Physical outcomes are clearly easier to measure. It is obvious that the patient's physical, social and emotional status will need to be taken into account, since this also influences the patient's outcome. However, there are at present few instruments available that measure outcome.

Table 1. Three interlocking components which affect care.

The three components interact. For example, we can see that the presence or absence of pressure sores could be an outcome measure of the quality of nursing care. But to say that the quality of nursing care is poor on Ward X because of the incidence of pressure sores would be unfair if we did not also take into account structural standards. It may be that the incidence of pressure sores has more to do with the patient's environmental condition than the type and frequency of nursing care; or it could be related to the lack of nursing staff or absence of equipment which means that the patients are not receiving the care prescribed.

What of the process component? To continue with the above example, pressure sores may develop in patients who are not debilitated and on wards judged to have sufficient staff or equipment. What type of nursing care have these patients been receiving? Is the nature of nursing care appropriate? Or may the nursing itself contribute to the incidence of pressure sores? This example illustrates the interrelationship of the components of evaluation or measurement of nursing care and also serves to demonstrate its complexity.

But the fact that something is complex is not an excuse for not tackling it. As referred to earlier, many of us are already collecting information that can be used in this type of framework. Structural aspects are most readily identifiable: eg the number of staff on the wards, the mix of different nursing grades among ward staff, the nature of patients' illnesses, the ward environment, and the availability of equipment. The list is endless. Some measures of the outcomes are also identifiable, such as: infection rates, letters of appreciation/complaint, numbers of deaths, discharges, and some physical conditions and behavioural activities. Outcomes can be measured by interviewing the patient and significant others, observation and auditing the patient's care plan.

Measurement of the process element of care is the one that has received the most attention. This is because process measures focus on what the nurse does. Such measurement implies that nursing is observable and controllable. However, any measurement of process should include the nurse's sensitivity and empathy for the patient and significant others. This is not easy to evaluate.

Tools for measuring quality of care
The tools available to measure quality attempt to draw together the components of evaluation already described above. While it is often tempting to develop one's own tool for measurement it is not always necessary to reinvent the wheel. It may be worthwhile considering and reviewing what is available. Each of the tools so far developed have their limitations but that does not invalidate their use given the immense complexity of their task. The better-known methods of measuring the quality of nursing care include: Rush/Medicus, Quality Patient Care Scale (Qualpac; Wandelt and Ager, 1984), and Phaneuf's Nursing Audit (1976) which were developed in the USA, and the Quality of Care Index (Monitor) which has been developed in the UK from the Rush/Medicus system (Figures 1 and 2).

Achieving a balance
Some readers may think that such a comprehensive approach as described is too time consuming and might detract from the provision of a high

```
        3.6  The Patient's Family is Included in the Nursing Care Process

3.601   IS THERE A WRITTEN STATEMENT WITH REGARD TO THE FAMILY'S LEVEL          No              1
        OF UNDERSTANDING, CONCERNS, OR VIEW OF THE PATIENT'S CONDITION?         Yes             2
                                                                               Not Applicable  3
            Applies to the past seven days.  Refers to responses
            probably elicited by question: 'LET'S DISCUSS SOME OF YOUR
            CONCERNS WITH REGARD TO MR _____'S CONDITION'.

            Look for documentation in patient record/Kardex.

3.602   DO THE NURSE, PATIENT AND FAMILY DISCUSS THE FAMILY'S                   No              1
        PARTICIPATION IN THE CARE OF THE PATIENT?                              Yes             2
                                                                               Not Applicable  3
            To patient four years and older: DOES YOUR FAMILY COME TO
            VISIT YOU?

            If yes, ask: IN THE PAST WEEK HAVE ANY OF THE NURSES TALKED
            WITH YOU AND YOUR FAMILY ABOUT WHAT THINGS THEY MIGHT HELP
            YOU DO?

            Refers to any assistance provided by the family.

3.603   IS OPPORTUNITY PROVIDED FOR FAMILY TO DISCUSS FEARS AND                 No              1
        ANXIETIES?                                                             Yes             2
                                                                               Not Applicable  3
            To nurse: HAVE MR _____'S FAMILY BEEN IN TO VISIT HIM IN
            THE PAST TWO DAYS?

            If patient has been on unit less than two days, ask:
            HAVE MR _____'S FAMILY BEEN IN TO VISIT HIM SINCE HE/SHE
            HAS BEEN HERE?

            If no, Code NA.

            If yes, ask nurse: HAVE ANY OF THE NURSES SPENT SOME TIME
            WITH THEM TO SEE IF THEY HAVE ANY PARTICULAR FEARS OR
            PROBLEMS RELATED TO MR _____'S ILLNESS?
```

Figure 1. Questionnaire sample from the Rush/Medicus system for quality assurance.

```
                              SECTION II

                  Source of Information:  Patient Observation


2.101   IS THE PATIENT WEARING AN IDENTIFICATION BRACELET OR TAG?               No              1
                                                                               Yes             2
            Patient must be wearing some form of identification bracelet or
            tag, even if not required by hospital policy.  Do not answer NA.


2.102   IS THE PATIENT IN A POSITION OF OPTIMAL BODY ALIGNMENT?                 No              1
                                                                               Yes             2
            Observe position of feet, legs, knees, trunk, shoulders, arms     Not Applicable  3
            and head.  Code No if any part of body not properly aligned.


2.103   ARE THE PATIENT'S NAILS CLEAN?                                          No              1
                                                                               Yes             2


2.104   IS THE PATIENT IN A POSITION FOR MAXIMAL LUNG EXPANSION?                No              1
                                                                               Yes             2
            Observe elevation of bed, use of pillows and position of head,     Not Applicable  3
            neck and chest.

            Answer Yes only if all indicators good.
```

Figure 2. Questionnaire sample from the Rush/Medicus system for quality assurance

quality of nursing care. Such criticisms are not new. As nurses, we are always ready to ask for something quick and easy. However, there are dangers in the quick and easy approach, since after a time the observations may be predicted and consequently the quality scores could be manipulated. Conversely, some methods do take a long time to administer and this can be exhausting for patients, staff, and those undertaking the measuring. If this is the case, the method or tool will lose credibility and nurses will be reluctant to use it. It is essential that a balance is achieved between comprehensiveness and ease of use.

Improving the quality of care

When the nursing care on the ward or in the unit has been monitored using one of these tools for measurement and a quality score established, what does it mean? How can it be used?

Ward staff should receive the results of the monitoring as soon as possible and these should be relayed to them in a positive and constructive manner. The score, in association with the information on numbers of staff available and the levels of dependency of patients, provides a basis for the ward sister and senior nurse to set standards of care for the future. They should agree the improvements to be made and the facilities and opportunities for further training necessary to make such improvements possible. In setting these standards and plans for future action, care must be taken to ensure that the targets are realistic and achievable. If quality assurance is to have meaning and if standards of care are to be improved, then those giving the care must be given the chance to succeed: they must be able to demonstrate that changes have taken place and that this is not simply another paper exercise.

Whichever instrument is developed or chosen, the senior managers must give positive support to the staff involved. This includes selecting the "right" people to do the measuring: people with a commitment to the improvement of quality, with clinical credibility, the ability to make objective judgements, and the ability to report accurately on what they see. This requires appropriate training and sound educational and training programmes are a necessary investment. Training is required not only for observers but also, perhaps more importantly, to meet the learning needs of staff, which may be identified as a result of measuring the quality of care.

As nurses, we may feel that such scientific approaches as proposed above are too far removed from the "art" of nursing. We must, however, combine the best of both the art and the science of nursing and utilize the very real talents that we have. If we do not, our very future as a profession may be endangered.

References

Donabedian, A. (1966) Some Issues in Evaluating the Quality of Nursing Care. *American Journal of Public Health*, **59,** 1833

Goldstone, L.A., Ball, J.A.., and Collier, M.M. (1983) *MONITOR – An Index of the Quality of Nursing Care for Acute Medical and Surgical Wards*, Newcastle-upon-Tyne Polytechnic Products Ltd.

Hegyvary, S.T. (1979). Nursing Process: The Basis for Evaluating the Quality of Nursing Care. *International Nursing Review*, **26;4,** 113

Kemp, N., Richardson, E. (1990). Quality Assurance in Nursing Practice. Butterworth Heineman, London.

Phaneuf, M.C. (1976) *The Nursing Audit – Self regulation in Nursing Practice*, 2nd edn. Appleton-Century Crofts, New York.

Wandelt, M.A. and Ager, J.W. (1984) *Quality Patient Care Scale*, Appleton-Century Crofts, New York.

23
Defining quality assurance

Lynn M. Dunne, MA, RGN, RCNT
Quality Assurance Adviser, Richmond, Twickenham and Roehampton Health Authority

The New Collins Concise English Dictionary (1985) defines as follows:

Quality: a distinguishing characteristic or attribute; the basic character or nature of something; a degree or standard of excellence; having or showing excellence or superiority.

Assurance: a statement or assertion intended to inspire confidence; freedom from doubt; certainty.

Standard: an accepted or approved example of something against which others are judged or measured; a principle of propriety, honesty and integrity; a level of excellence or quality; of recognised authority, competence or excellence.

Monitor: to check (the technical quality of); a person or piece of equipment that warns, checks or keeps a continuous record of something.

Quality of nursing care embodies a certain degree of abstraction. It expresses reality and yet is also synonymous with aspects of desirability. Making the necessary distinction is often difficult especially in relation to individuals, as judgements may be clouded by subjectivity due to individual beliefs, values, expectations and cultural background. To overcome this problem it is suggested that effectiveness of care is measured using specific criteria, statements of performance, behaviour or circumstances (standards), derived from broad goals (values), which represent the views of the department and are acceptable to all concerned.

First nursing standards

The current wave of interest in nursing, quality assurance began in the early '80s. However the idea itself of measuring the quality and effectiveness of nursing care is not at all new. From 1854 to 1870 Florence Nightingale led the impetus for systematic evaluation of both the process of nursing care and its outcome in terms of patient wellbeing. When she and her team of nurses arrived at the Barrack Hospital, Scutari in 1854 the mortality rate was 32 per cent, within six months the mortality rate had fallen to aproximately two per cent, arguably the best performance indicator for the effectiveness of her nursing care.

Florence Nightingale also established what might be described as the first nursing standards in *Notes on Nursing* (Nightingale, 1860), in which she stated that the first rule of the hospital was that it should do the patient no harm. The book went on to describe the importance and benefits of cleanliness and fresh air for patients and underlined the need to prevent overcrowding in hospitals to control infection amongst patients. This point is still relevant today, as many hospitals continue the practice of 'hot-bedding' for daycases. Nightingale also highlighted the importance of nurses being able to observe patients keenly, so that they might detect and report changes in a patient's condition. (Quite apart from the educational ramifications, how often is this point taken into consideration when designing new hospitals?)

Establishing quality assurance programmes

Efforts to establish quality assurance programmes began in 1918 in the USA. Rapid growth and development of nursing quality assurance activity took place there throughout the seventies and interest reached Britain towards the end of the decade. This was reflected by the publication of two discussion documents, 'Standards of Nursing Care' (RCN, 1980) and 'Towards Standards' (RCN, 1981), by the Royal College of Nursing.

Characteristics of quality

The two documents attempted to identify the characteristics of high quality nursing care. 'Standards of Nursing Care' (RCN, 1980), addressed the question "what constitutes good nursing care?", and the committee agreed that both the process and the outcome of nursing care should be taken into consideration and that by using collective professional judgement it would be possible to determine whether or not good nursing care had taken place. Good nursing care was defined as being planned, systematic and focused on the individual. The nursing process must obviously be used to evaluate the quality of nursing care.

Evaluating quality

There are now numerous tools available to evaluate the quality of nursing care in various clinical settings. It is still helpful to take one step further back and consider the model or framework from which a quality assurance programme can be developed. Figures 1 and 2 illustrate the models of quality assurance used by the American Nurses' Association and the Registered Nurses' Association of British Columbia, Canada. Both take a similar approach.

The first step in any quality assurance programme is to identify values and a philosophy/ideology for the department and individuals concerned. These will act as the cornerstone for the programme. In America and Canada this means a printed statement (often referred to as a mission statement) that can be found in every nursing office and ward. The mission statement clearly outlines what nursing (in that particular hospital/clinical setting) will and will not do. The next stage is the identification and formulation (writing) of valid, acceptable nursing

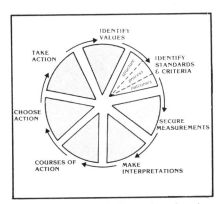

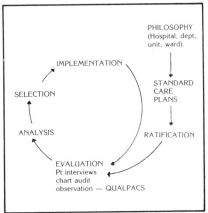

Figure 1. Adapted from the American Nurses' Association model for quality assurance programmes.

Figure 2. The Registered Nurses' Association of British Columbia model for quality assurance.

standards (in Canada these were expressed in standard care plan format as opposed to a list of formal statements which is more popular in the USA). These standards cover such areas as nursing manpower levels, equipment, clinical practice, nurse education (ie ward learning climate) and patient responses to the nursing care delivered.

Evaluating present practice

Having agreed upon their standards the nursing department's next step is to measure present practice against the desired, pre-set standard to determine whether or not the service provided is acceptable or whether some form of remedial action and in-service education needs to be taken. The appropriate course of action is then selected and implemented and the problem/remedial action reassessed to see whether or not the problem has been resolved. Should further action be required, intervention takes place at the appropriate stage of the quality assurance model. Thus the cycle of quality monitoring is continuous, aiming to consistently improve or maintain a high standard of nursing care.

There are three common approaches that can be taken when developing a system to monitor the quality of nursing practice:

Prospective approach To a certain extent this type of assessment is something of a paradox. You may well be wondering how care can be evaluated before it is given. In reality prospective quality monitoring tends to be the prior identification of types or groups of patients — ie the next 20 patients admitted who are deemed to be at risk from developing pressure sores using the Norton Score (Norton, 1975). Once the patients have been identified evaluation of their care will take place either concurrently or retrospectively.

Concurrent approach   This is an evaluation procedure that takes place while the patient is still in hospital. It tends to focus on the quality of the nursing actions themselves (the process of nursing) and involves direct observation of nurses giving care, questioning patients and chart audit. An obvious benefit to this method is that information can be used to improve a patient's care while he or she is still in hospital should it be found wanting in any respect.

Retrospective approach   A review of care that takes place after a patient has been discharged from hospital. Audits of patient records and charts is the most usual method. Obviously this approach does not have the benefits of concurrent studies (influencing care whilst the patient is still in hospital) but it does allow a comprehensive evaluation of the whole case to take place. Valuable information can be gained about successful nursing care that staff would wish to repeat and likewise unsuccessful nursing intervention that staff should avoid in future.

Whatever method is chosen, the emphasis should be on solving known or suspected problems revealed by the monitoring process which affect patient care or the nursing service detrimentally and cannot be justified.

The quality assurance programme may be designed by an individual or an elected committee but it is important that it is owned and accepted by the staff implementing nursing care to patients. Including some or all of the staff involved in patient care areas (depending on the size of the hospital) in developing the programme would certainly provide a broader perspective and hopefully increase commitment and participation.

Thorough planning

Thorough planning is essential to strengthen and secure the programme and allow participants to be directed and supported.

Many nurses harbour negative feelings towards quality assurance programmes. They are often suspicious of management's motives for such an exercise, fearing cost cutting measures. There is a certain reluctance among the profession to review the care given to patients (as can be seen in its failure to get to grips with evaluation of planned patient care since the adoption of the nursing process by the General Nursing Council in 1977), and personal performance. This is hardly surprising in a system where few hospitals even today practise employee appraisal. It may help to point out to staff that they are already carrying out some quality monitoring activities, nearly all clinical areas have some form of quality control (infection control, review of domestic services), thus proving that quality assurance is not such an alien and theoretical topic.

It is important to distinguish between quality assurance and quality monitoring/control (Figure 3). Quality monitoring is a crucial part of any quality assurance programme and is the process whereby current practice is compared with pre-determined standards. It is however not quality assurance (freedom from doubt concerning the degree of excellence).

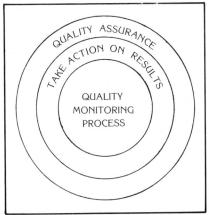

Figure 3. The relationship (and difference) between the quality monitoring process and quality assurance adapted with kind permission from Lang (1974).

Quality assurance is only present when current nursing practice has been compared with the standard and appropriate action has been taken successfully to remedy the problems identified.

Running quality assurance programmes

Staff frequently need help to realise that unless action is taken on the results of quality control and monitoring, then quality assurance cannot be achieved (Figure 3). Involving ward staff in developing the programme and utilising their experience and skills by asking them to act as assessors/ observers is important in overcoming negative feelings and running a meaningful programme. Management must be committed to replacing any staff taken away from clinical areas to participate in the programme, or to pay the necessary overtime.

Quality assurance programmes should only deal with problems that will have a positive effect on patient care or nursing practice when resolved and which can be remedied within existing, available resources (realistic problem solving). Likewise, the prioritising of problems will depend on their effects on patient care and resources. The causes of selected problems must be identified and options outlined for action. Finally the programme must include documentation of problem resolution and indicate to what extent the desired change has been achieved.

The completed quality assurance manual should be available in all nursing departments, with the relevant evaluation reports and action plans. Improvements and problem resolution should be noted and praised and management should be quick to highlight staff who have made particular efforts in this direction. Feedback and knowledge of results regarding a department's quality assessment should be as fast as possible to maintain staff motivation and commitment.

The aim of every nurse and nursing service is surely to provide the highest quality nursing care possible given the presenting situation and resources. It therefore follows that each nursing service must strive to develop a quality assurance programme that accurately measures the level of goal attainment within its clinical areas. To design a successful programme, time must be spent planning well defined goals and objectives, reviewing existing activities that attempt to measure quality and building on them with the cooperation of nursing staff at all levels.

References

Lang, N. (1974) A model for quality assurance in nursing. In: *A Plan for Implementation of Standards of Nursing Practice*. Kansas City Mo: ANA 1975.

Nightingale, F. (1860) *Notes on Nursing*. Dover Publications Inc., 1969, New York, USA.

Norton, D. (1975) *An Investigation of Geriatric Nursing Problems in Hospital*. Churchill Livingstone, Edinburgh.

Royal College of Nursing (1980) *'Standards of Nursing Care'* a discussion document. RCN, London.

Royal College of Nursing (1981) *'Towards Standards'* – a discussion document. RCN, London.

Bibliography

Meisenheimer, C.G. (1985). *Quality Assurance: a complete guide to effective programmes*. (1st edition). Aspen Systems Corporation, USA.
   Bought in USA, may be difficult to obtain in the UK.

24

How do we set nursing standards?

Lynn M. Dunne, MA, RGN, RCNT
Quality Assurance Adviser, Richmond, Twickenham and Roehampton Health Authority

Nursing standards are valid, acceptable definitions of the quality of nursing care, and cannot be valid unless they contain a means of measuring (criteria) to enable nursing care to be evaluated in terms of effectiveness and quality. When standards are written without criteria (eg 'the patient will not suffer postoperative pain'), the effect is similar to using a ruler without measurements marked on when making a scale drawing. The measurements would have to be guessed, would undoubtedly be wildly inaccurate and they would certainly vary enormously from one individual to another (Mason, 1978).

Implicit in Florence Nightingale's famous statement that the first requirement of a hospital is that it should do the patient no harm (Strauss, 1967) is the idea that nursing care should be of a high standard and through her continued scrutiny of nursing practice she strove to attain this goal. More recently in the UK the Royal College of Nursing, concerned with the promotion of nursing and the ability of its members to provide and maintain an adequate standard of care to their patients, published two authoritative documents on setting, monitoring and evaluating standards of care within the nursing profession (RCN, 1980; RCN, 1981).

What is nursing care?
It is important that before trying to evaluate their individual or collective performances, nurses should have a clear understanding of what 'nursing' and 'nursing care' actually mean. Nursing departments can accept a well known definition of nursing such as 'The unique function of the nurse is to assist the individual, sick or well, in the performance of those activities contributing to health and its recovery (or to a peaceful death), that he would perform unaided if he had the necessary strength, will or knowledge; and to do this in such a way as to help him gain independence as rapidly as possible' (Henderson, 1979). Alternatively they can opt for an in-house definition (mission statement) (Dunne, 1986) that has been ratified by the nursing staff. Which they accept is purely a matter of choice, but it must reflect the values of the nursing service concerned.

The concept of nursing care standards is immediately complicated as the phrase becomes synonymous with both the quality and effectiveness of care. The word 'standards' has both qualitative and quantitative connotations, it may be something that serves as a basis for comparison (a yardstick) or a measure of the level of performance (output) required of an individual. Previous studies of the effectiveness of nursing care have concentrated on the quantitative aspects; however current emphasis is on a more holistic approach, attempting to evaluate the more discrete qualitative issues in nursing care eg interpersonal and communication skills.

'Standards of Nursing Care' (RCN, 1980) suggests that the most suitable method of deciding what constitutes good nursing care is by identifying desired nursing behaviours. Observation of current nursing practice and comparison with predetermined standards would enable nurses to judge whether or not good nursing care had taken place. The report defines desired nursing behaviour as being planned, purposeful, systematic and goal directed, ie the use of the nursing process. 'Towards Standards' (RCN, 1981), in considering how to formulate nursing standards, felt that the writing of checklists, norms and ratios was inappropriate and instead identified eight key factors for professional nursing standards (Table 1).

1. A philosophy of nursing.
2. The relevant knowledge and skills.
3. The nurse's authority to act.
4. Accountability.
5. The control of resources.
6. The organisational structure and management style.
7. The doctor/nurse relationship.
8. The management of change.

Table 1. Prerequisites for the professional control of standards of nursing care.

Accountability

Of these eight factors, accountability is the most central to the formation of professional standards. Nurses must also be clear about the extent of their authority, and responsibility and accountability must be matched with the necessary authority to carry out the job effectively. Senior nurses must be prepared to provide the nurse with the tools to do the job — ie manpower, equipment. Devolving accountability to individual nurses may well be the long term answer to improving standards of nursing care but the profession should ask itself if this move is really appropriate now, in a system that still entrusts the majority of its 'basic care' to untrained/unqualified individuals?

Having looked at what nursing standards are and the key areas related to them, how do we set these standards? In his review of the evaluation of the quality of medical care, Avedis Donabedian outlined three approaches (studying the structural variables, studying the process of care and reviewing the outcome of care in patients); these approaches are still widely used by nurses in the field of quality assurance, as most areas of nursing fall into one or more of the three categories (Donabedian, 1966). The three categories when applied to evaluating the quality of nursing care may be defined as follows:

Structure standards   These regulate nursing practice and include the organisation of nursing services, recruitment, selection, manpower establishments, provision of necessary equipment, buildings and include all the processes of licensing, eg National Board educational visits to approve facilities for learner/post basic education. They generally tend to indicate minimum expectations or levels of service, eg there will always be at least one RGN on duty on the ward at all times.

Process standards   These look specifically at the actions performed by nurses and define the quality of the implementation of nursing care. Nursing departments should develop process standards for all nursing interventions (nursing procedures). Nursing procedures and process standards, although similar, are not the same thing.

Outcome standards   The patient's response to planned care, ie the expected change in a patient's condition following nursing intervention, is an outcome standard. Nursing action may result in positive or negative outcomes for a patient (positive outcomes being beneficial and appropriate nursing intervention, and negative outcomes inappropriate nursing care). Outcome standards frequently include some measure of the patient's satisfaction with the care. Many authors define a further category:

Content standards   These describe the nature of nursing that is communicated to other groups or disciplines and the basis of nursing decisions, ie information that must be recorded in nursing notes and reported to the multidisciplinary team, communication and teaching of patients and their families or friends (Mason, 1978).

Writing standards

Many standards set for a nursing service will concern clinical work (direct nursing care given to patients), and tend to be written in the form of principles of nursing practice (the foundation of but not quite as detailed as a nursing procedure). The seven steps outlined below can be used when writing any nursing standard (structure, process, outcome or content); here they are illustrated using the example of the process standards set for performing endotracheal suction of a ventilated patient.

1. Select the area of nursing for which the standard is to be written and identify the type (structure, process, outcome, content) eg **process standard:** endotracheal suction of a ventilated patient.

2. Identify the objectives for the standard stating explicitly what you intend to achieve. The objectives may be nurse centred or patient centred:

Nurse-centred objectives
a. To apply suction to the patient without introducing infection into the respiratory tract.
b. To prevent trauma to the respiratory tract.

Patient-centred objectives
c. The patient will not experience hypoxia during the suction procedure, ie PO_2 of no less than 11kPa.
d. The patient will not experience anxiety or distress during the suction procedure.

3. Specify the nursing action essential to achieve the objectives, eg:
a. Wash your hands; use sterile equipment and an aseptic technique.
b. Apply suction only when withdrawing catheter.
c. Hyperoxygenate patient prior to the procedure (if prescribed) with ventilator or re-breathing bag for one minute prior to suction procedure.
d. Do not apply suction for more than 15 seconds; suction only until secretions are removed.

4. Where possible specify a time frame for each action, eg apply suction for no more than 15 seconds.

5. Write up the standard in a logical order, eg i. Define subject. ii. Identify objectives. iii. List standards.

6. Review the work done to eliminate ambiguous or irrelevant information that cannot be evaluated, eg suggestions for procedure technique.

7. Test the new standard for acceptability and validity.

Who should write the standards?

In order to decide who should write these standards, it is useful to identify the size of the task, the types of standards to be written and the resources available, eg nurse managers, educationalists and clinical specialists, and to use them as effectively as possible. It is essential that the meaning of any nursing standard is shared, accepted and understood by those who have written it and those expected to implement it.

Examples of nursing standards that should be found currently in any hospital would include a nursing practice and policy manual that is based on current nursing research findings, the use of specific ward learning outcomes for learner nurses in ward areas, the practice of individualised patient care through the use of the nursing process, adherence to National Board training requirements, staff ratios of trained staff: learners and compliance with the UKCC code of professional conduct.

Location of standards

Once written, all nursing standards should be easily accessed and referred to by the nursing staff either before, during or after nursing intervention. Formulating and measuring nursing standards is not akin to setting a closed book exam or an attempt to catch individuals out, so it is only right and proper that staff should know what is expected of them before their action and its effects on patients are critically evaluated on either a collective or individual basis.

High quality nursing care does not happen by accident, it must be planned for and evaluated against pre-set standards so that nurses can recognise and repeat good nursing care and avoid mistakes in the future (McFarlane, 1979).

Nurses have a responsibility to society, themselves and their colleagues in the health care services to ensure they provide the highest quality care possible in the presenting situation and resources. Nursing standards are the key to any successful quality assurance programme as they define valid, acceptable, measurable levels of performance and outcome against which current nursing practice must and will be judged and evaluated.

References

Donabedian, A. (1966) Evaluating the quality of medical care. *Millbank Memorial Fund Quarterly*, **4,** 166–203.

Dunne, L. (1986) Developing quality assurance. *The Professional Nurse*, **2,** 2, 47–9.

Henderson, V. (2979) *Basic Principles of Nursing Care.* (11th edition). International Council of Nurses. Geneva, Switzerland.

McFarlane, J.K. (1979) Take aim and shoot for goal. *Nursing Mirror.* (supplement). 19.4.79. xx-xxviii.

Mason, E.J. (1978) *How to Write Meaningful Nursing Standards.* (2nd edition) John Wiley and Sons Inc, USA.

NB Bought in USA. J. Wiley outlets in UK.

Royal College of Nursing, (1980) *'Standards of Nursing Care' – a discussion document.* RCN, London.

Royal College of Nursing, (1981) *'Towards Standards' – a discussion document.* RCN, London.

Strauss, M.B. (1967) *Familiar Medical Quotations.* (1st edition) J.A. Churchill Ltd, London.

25

Qualpacs: a practical guide

Paul Wainwright, SRN, MSc, DANS, DipN, RNT
Professional Adviser, Welsh National Board for Nursing, Midwifery and Health Visiting

There are several quality monitoring tools available to nurses, including Quality Patient Care Scale, also known as Qualpacs (Wandelt and Ager, 1974). We shall discuss here some of the practical problems involved in putting Qualpacs to work in the ward.

Commitment

The first point to be clear about if you want to measure the quality of care in your area of practice, with Qualpacs or any other tool, is that you and your colleagues really want to do it. To ask nurses to expose their practice to observation and criticism by others is asking a lot, and if there is no commitment to look constructively at the result, the whole exercise will be pointless. The decision to use any quality measuring tool should only be taken after thorough discussion with all the staff involved, including the area manager. An involved and supportive manager is an invaluable ally, who may be able to provide material help with things like photocopying, typing, or extra cover for a meeting of all the ward staff. He or she may offer moral support, share some of the risks and offer a different perspective if things get difficult. The manager may also be able to put you in touch with other helpers, perhaps someone in the school or at district headquarters, who you may not know about. You may even have a standards officer or quality assurance manager to whom you can go for help.

Is Qualpacs the tool for you?

Having thrashed out such questions as: ''do we really want to measure quality and why?'' and: ''what are we going to do with the results of our measurements?'', you can think about which tool to use. Perhaps the most important task at this stage is to decide what quality nursing means to you and your colleagues. Unless you are sure of your values you cannot begin to set standards or measure quality.

If your ward or team has not got a written statement of your nursing philosophy, with some statements about beliefs and values, this is the first step. Measuring quality is a subjective business, involving choices. If no-one agrees beforehand what their preferences are, the result would be like organising a night out at the local Indian restaurant and expecting everyone to enjoy the food, even though nobody else but you likes spices.

Preparing the ground

Assuming you have a philosophy which everyone supports, the next job is to read everything you can find about tools in general. The bibliography at the end of this chapter will help.

Qualpacs involves watching the care being given, as well as some consideration of charts and records and other aspects of communication. It attaches great importance to individual patient care and involvement and expects the nurse to have good interpersonal skills. If you and your colleagues share these values, Qualpacs may well be the tool for you. However, be wary of measuring only the things you think you are good at. You may get a shock if you find out you are not as good as you thought (which is a good thing to know), but you may also be tempted not to look at things where you know you are weak.

If all the nurse-patient interaction in your area is excellent, but the standard of record keeping is poor you might be well advised to use a chart audit of some sort, either instead of, or as well as, Qualpacs.

Validity and reliability

The concepts of validity and reliability are discussed briefly in Figure 1. You will also find a more detailed discussion in the text of Qualpacs and in Barnett and Wainwright (1987).

Subjectivity: If I stand at the end of the bed and look at a patient I may form all sorts of impressions and opinions about him, but these will be subjective judgements based on my experience, knowledge, beliefs and values. Indeed, to say: subjective judgements, is tautology, since judgements are by definition subjective. Much of the work of any profession is based on subjectivity, because no matter how many hard facts you may possess about something, you will always have to exercise judgement when deciding what to do about it. This is not something to be ashamed or frightened of. It is simply a matter of recognising the importance of professional judgement and making sure that it is based on as much good evidence as possible.

Objectivity: The opposite of subjectivity. An accurate thermometer correctly used will give an objective measure of body temperature. No opinion or judgement comes into it.

Validity: To say that a measure is valid is to say that it actually measures what it claims (or is being used) to measure. Thus a clock can give a valid measurement of time and a thermometer can give a valid measurement of temperature.

Reliability: A reliable instrument is one which gives the same result consistently if it is used repeatedly to measure the same thing, by the same or by different people. If a thermometer records a patient's temperature as being sometimes a degree more than it really is, and sometimes a degree less, then it is not reliable. Neither is the clock which sometimes gains and sometimes loses. Of course, some tools may give different results depending who is using them. It is important that all users agree to use the same methods, otherwise the results will be unreliable through no fault of the tool. A tool may be reliable, but not valid, as for example a clock which is always ten minutes fast.

Figure 1. Definitions of subjectivity, objectivity, validity and reliability.

Having decided you want to use Qualpacs, the next thing to do is to read the items in the questionnaire and the cues once again. This time you and your colleagues need to ask yourselves: "do we really understand what this item means? How will we recognise this behaviour when we see it, and what represents good and bad performance?" I would advise you not to alter the wording of any of the items in the questionnaire, but you are at liberty to make minor alterations or additions to the cues that go with it. This will enable you to give examples that relate to your area of practice. It will also ensure that everyone in the team has the same understanding of the items.

At this stage, if you have not already done so, you will have to decide who are to be the observers who will carry out the exercise. There is no rule about this, other than that they must be practising nurses who know something about your area of work and, above all, are acceptable to the staff to be monitored. An adverse report is easily rationalised away if it can be suggested that the observers did not know what they were looking at. The observers could be members of staff in the area concerned who will monitor their colleagues at work, from another similar area, from a neighbouring unit, hospital or district, managers, teaching staff, or anybody else who is acceptable, available and willing. Preparing for and carrying out the exercise will require some commitment and time from the observers, so you may need to negotiate with the relevant managers, to release them from duties or provide cover for them.

Training the observers

The observers will then have to be trained to use the tool. This does not take long, perhaps three days in total, but will require some organisation. A friendly tutor or helpful in-service department could be invaluable. Training should include:

- introducing the concept of quality measurement;
- introducing Qualpacs;
- giving everyone time to read through the items and cues;
- discussion of the concepts of validity, reliability and objectivity;
- discussion of the items and cues so that everyone understands and agrees them;
- discussion of the five point, best-nurse-poorest-nurse scale;
- discussion of practical problems — where to sit when observing, how to cope with rapid activities, ensuring privacy and so on;
- practice sessions in clinical areas other than the one to be monitored;
- debriefing sessions to compare scores and establish reliability.

The objective of the practice sessions is that if two or more observers watch the same patients getting the same care without comparing notes at the time, when their scores are checked afterwards they should be very close to each other. The Qualpacs text discusses this and suggests the degree of correlation that should be obtained. If you are not sure about things like correlation coefficients you can probably find a statistician in your district headquarters, or the school of nursing, or at a local college, who will help.

Many modern scientific calculators have a correlation function built in, which makes life simpler. If, having done all this you find your observers produce very different scores, they need to sit down together and go over their notes from the session, comparing their responses to the various situations and finding out where they differed. They should then repeat the exercise and check that their scores are now close enough to be acceptable.

Rating the procedures

The trickiest thing for newcomers to using tools like Qualpacs is the concentration needed to watch a nurse do something, split it up into four or five different components, find those items in the questionnaire, and rate how well they were done. For example, while bathing a patient, a nurse may pay attention to him, treat him in a kind and friendly manner, choose appropriate topics for conversation, utilise the nursing procedure as an opportunity for patient interaction, give the patient information, respond appropriately to him, observe changes in his condition and react accordingly, adapt the procedure to meet his needs, involve him in decision making, record information about him or communicate it to others, as well as maintaining his privacy and dignity and observing acceptable standards of hygiene and cleanliness and making him feel safe!

All of these (and more) are noted separately in Qualpacs, and the same nurse may do them well one minute and poorly the next, with the same patient. She may also change from patient to patient. However, with practice it is possible to record a surprising amount of detail with great accuracy.

Using the tool

It is essential to plan ahead and make sure everyone involved in the project knows what is happening. You will probably have discussed the project with your manager at intervals, but have a final session to go through all the arrangements. Pick an ordinary day: you are not trying to prove how hard you work or how short staffed you are, so don't choose the morning when there are three lists and two ward rounds all at the same time. Pick the patients to be monitored, randomly if possible, though the final choice will be partly governed by their condition, the layout of the ward, and their willingness to take part. Explain to the patients what is going to happen and ask their permission. Explain what is happening to other staff — domestics, porters and doctors — so that they are not worried by the sight of people with clip-boards busily writing down everything that happens. Don't be afraid to cancel at the last minute if unforseen problems crop up. Introduce the observers to the patients and make sure that everyone knows they are observers, and that they cannot help with care or do anything for patients except in dire emergency.

The report

There is no point in spending a lot of time and effort — and therefore money — on an exercise like Qualpacs if you don't intend to use the findings. There must be a commitment from the start to respond constructively to criticism and use the report as the basis for change and improvement. Nevertheless, the staff will have found the experience of being observed quite uncomfortable and will be apprehensive about the outcome. A useful tactic to prepare for the feedback session is to ask the staff to jot down the points they think are going to come out in the report.

Most people have a reasonable degree of insight into their strengths and weaknesses, and will probably err on the critical side if asked to appraise themselves. It should then prove possible to start the feedback with the positive aspects, and you may be able to say of the bad points: ''it was better than you expected, though there is room for improvement''. People are much more likely to accept that they have faults and to look for remedies if they have identified the faults themselves, and have the opportunity to find their own solutions.

A serious undertaking

Measuring the quality of care in your area is not a task to undertake lightly. This article has touched on many of the problems, but has deliberately skimmed the surface in many areas, assuming that you will get hold of Qualpacs and some of the many other articles about it, and read this article in conjunction with them. I do strongly recommend that you seek help from people you trust and spend a lot of time preparing and planning before you do anything. That said, if you wish to recognise your professional responsibility to evaluate the quality of what you do, I wish you well!

References

Barnett, D. Wainwright, P.J. (1987) A measure of quality. *Senior Nurse*, **6**, 3, 8–9.
Dunne, L.M. (1987) Quality Assurance: methods of measurement. *The Professional Nurse*, **26**, 187–190.
Wandelt, M. and Ager, J. (1974) Quality Patient Care Scale (QUALPACS). Appleton Century Crofts, New York.

Bibliography

Barnett, D. and Wainwright P.J. (1987) Between two tools. *Senior Nurse*, **6**, 4, 40–2.
Barnett, D. and Wainwright P.J. (1987) The right reflection. *Senior Nurse*, **6**, 5, 33–34.
Burford Nursing Development Unit. (1983-84) A compendium of articles published in British nursing journals by staff at BNDU. Available on application to SNDU, Burford, Oxfordshire.
Burnip, S. and Wainwright, P.J. (1983) Qualpacs at Burford. *Nursing Times*, 36–38.
Dunne, L.M. (1987) How do we set nursing standards? *The Professional Nurse*, **2**, 4, 107–9.
Kemp, N. (1986) What is quality assurance? *The Professional Nurse*, **1**, 5, 124–126.
Kitson, A.L. (1986) Indicators of quality in nursing care: an alternative approach. *Journal of Advanced Nursing*, **11**, 133–144.
Kitson, A.L. and Kendall, H. (1986) Rest assured. *Nursing Times*, 29–31.

Kitson, A.L. (1986) Taking action. *Nursing Times*, 52–54.
Wainwright, P.J. (1987) Peer review: in Pearson, A. (Ed), Nursing Quality Measurement, 15–24. John Wiley and Sons.
Wilson-Barnett, J. (1986) A measure of care. *Nursing Times*, 57–58.

26

Quality assurance: methods of measurement

Lynn M. Dunne, MA, RGN, RCNT

Quality Assurance Adviser, Richmond, Twickenham and Roehampton Health Authority

Attempts to define quality assurance (Dunne, 1986) and how a nursing service might set acceptable standards of nursing care (Dunne, 1987), have already been made. In the next phase a method of measuring current nursing practice against pre-determined standards must be developed. The four methods reviewed here: Qualpacs, Nursing Audit (Phaneuf), the Rush-Medicus System and Monitor, are among several currently available.

Qualpacs

The Quality Patient Care Scale (Qualpacs) was developed by Mabel Wandelt and Joel Ager at the College of Nursing, Wayne State University, Michigan, USA in the early 1970s, a time that saw a rapid increase in knowledge and literature about quality assurance in North America.

It is a tool based on evaluation of the *process* of nursing (ie how nursing care is delivered to patients), by direct observation. The scale itself lists 68 items of nursing care, arranged under six subsections as follows:

Psychosocial: Individual Actions directed towards meeting the psychosocial needs of individual patients.

Psychosocial: Group Actions directed towards meeting the psychosocial needs of patients as members of a group.

Physical: Actions directed towards meeting physical needs.

General: Actions that may be directed toward meeting either psychosocial or physical needs of the patient or both at the same time.

Communication: Communication on behalf of the patient.

Professional implications: Care given to patients reflects initiative and responsibility indicative of professional expectations.

Two or more trained observers evaluate all interaction between nurses and patients in a clinical area for two hours. Any one of the 68 items is scored on a scale of one to five (Table 1).

Wandelt and Ager advocate that Qualpacs observers complete an orientation programme which allows sufficient time for them to become familiar with the background to the Qualpacs; the cue sheets for each section, individual items and spend some time (two days is suggested) discussing what standards are acceptable and becoming familiar with the

```
1 = Poorest care
2 = Between
3 = Average care (that expected of
    a newly qualified RGN)
4 = Between
5 = Best care
```

Table 1. Qualpacs scoring method.

actual use of the rating scale.

The use of Qualpacs evokes a mixed response from nurses. Those who are against it express doubts about the tool as a reliable, objective method, saying it is both subjective (as it is the opinion of the observer as to whether poor, average or best care has taken place and that is highly dependent on previous experience and personal values). The counter argument to this is simple: if you reject Qualpacs on the basis that it is subjective and therefore unreliable it is tantamount to saying you reject the professional judgement of nurses in matters related to nursing practice (for previous experience and personal values are the basis of professional judgement also), which in turn opens Pandora's Box on such issues as the necessity to have a nurse(s) in charge of nursing.

Many groups and individuals (particularly trade unions) fear that as Qualpacs looks at individual nurses and the care they give to patients, the opportunity exists to use the findings in a disciplinary manner if poor or unsafe practice is observed. Certain steps can be taken to overcome these potential problems. First, only nurses with a clinical involvement should order a Qualpacs assessment or act as observers and second, feedback should be direct between the observers and the ward nurses. Management should not have access to a Qualpacs assessment as part of an investigation or disciplinary procedure. This approach has been used successfully at Burford Nursing Development Unit and is now used throughout Oxfordshire Health Authority.

In its favour it must be said that as a direct observation tool, Qualpacs provides an opportunity to improve care and benefit patients while they are still in hospital. Many people involved in quality assurance feel that direct observation of nursing care is the most effective way of evaluating its quality and is critical to the success of any quality assurance programme.

The Phaneuf Nursing Audit
This audit was developed by Maria Phaneuf in the mid 1970s and, as the name suggests, is an audit of nursing care taken from the patients' notes. Phaneuf herself described nursing audit as a process orientated approach to appraise the nursing process as reflected in the patients' records.

The Nursing Audit reviews 50 separate criteria which are grouped under seven headings as follows:
1. The application and execution of the doctor's legal orders.

2. The observation of symptoms and reactions.
3. Supervision of the patient.
4. Supervision of those participating in care (except the doctor).
5. Reporting and recording.
6. Application and execution of nursing procedures and techniques.
7. Promotion of physical and emotional health by direction and teaching.

The first part of the nursing audit consists of a patient details form (similar to many hospital admissions slips) which Phaneuf suggests can be completed by a member of clerical staff, eg ward clerk, as professional nursing knowledge is not required. The second part of the nursing audit is the evaluation of the patients care using his/her inpatient notes. The criteria are evaluated using yes/no/uncertain categories and scored accordingly. To arrive at the final score the total of the individual component scores is multiplied by the value of the 'does not apply' scores. The quality of nursing care is described in Table 2.

Score		Quality of Care
0 — 40	=	Unsafe
41 — 80	=	Poor
81 — 120	=	Incomplete .
121 — 160	=	Good
161 — 200	=	Excellent

Table 2. The Phaneuf Nursing Audit Scoring Method.

Nursing Audit has been widely criticised by many nurses who argue that nurses frequently give care that is not documented and conversely often document care that is never given to the patient. I suggest this somewhat cynical view of nursing practice is neither a typical nor fair representation, despite the profession's many faults, and that Nursing Audit has a useful role to play in evaluating quality as it is quick, simple and comprehensive. Familiarisation and training for assessors is easy too. The biggest barrier to using Nursing Audit in the UK is documentation as audit is only feasible in clinical areas using a systematic approach.

Many feel that Nursing Audit can be a useful part of a quality assurance programme. Burford Nursing Development Unit have successfully combined Qualpacs and Nursing Audit in their quality assurance programme (to overcome the criticisms of using each method independently) thus enabling nursing care to be evaluated as it is given to patients and retrospectively via the nursing records.

Rush Medicus System
The Rush-Medicus System was also a product of the early 70s (1972) and was the result of a collaborative project between the Medicus Systems Corporation and Rush Presbyterian St Luke's Medical Centre in Chicago and the Baptist Medical Centre in Birmingham, Alabama.

The conceptual framework chosen for the system was the Nursing Process which had been implemented at Rush Presbyterian St Luke's Medical Centre and the concept of patient needs. The nursing process was defined as the comprehensive set of nursing activities performed in the delivery of a patient's care; assessment of the problems or needs of the patient, planning for care, implementing the plan of care and evaluating/updating the plan of care.

It was hoped to develop a system that would evaluate all these areas. The concept was further enhanced by evaluating whether patient needs were actually being met in accordance with the care plan.

Once the conceptual framework was decided it had to be broken into logical components. Six objectives and 32 sub-objectives were outlined, which the project team believed defined the nursing care process succintly and with a degree of detail not achieved in previous programmes. The next step was to develop criteria that would evaluate each of the sub-objectives. A total of 357 criteria were developed (Master Criteria List).

The Master Criteria List is held on a computer programme which will produce up to 76 different questionnaires that can be used for patients in accident and emergency departments, labour and delivery wards, psychiatry, nursery, recovery and general medicine and surgery, according to their dependency group. In addition there are nine questionnaires which can be used for the parents of babies in the nursery and 18 ward based questionnaires that can be used in all clinical areas.

Ward areas tend to be evaluated three-to-four times per year in hospitals using the Rush-Medicus System in the USA. Quality monitoring takes place over a calendar month during which 10 per cent of the patient throughput is sampled.

Patients forming part of the quality assessment are selected using a random number table and their permission is then obtained verbally before proceeding. Nurse observers tend to be either staff nurses working at ward level who have completed the necessary observer's training course and belong to the hospital nursing quality assurance observers 'bank', or a small permanent team of observers who carry out all the nursing quality monitoring for the whole hospital.

The Rush-Medicus System has the advantage of having been extensively tested during its development (19 hospitals across the USA). It is now widely used by many hundreds of hospitals throughout the USA and Canada which form a users group that feeds in results to provide comparative scores and allows the tool to be updated. The disadvantages of the system are that it is large and time consuming to administer (most hospitals using Rush-Medicus have a full/part time coordinator) and a computer is a prerequisite to run the programme effectively.

Monitor
Of all the quality assurance systems mentioned in this chapter Monitor is probably the most familiar. It was developed by Goldstone, Ball and

Collier, (1984) as part of the North West Region Staffing Levels Project and is the adaptation for the UK of the Rush-Medicus System.

Monitor consists of four patient questionnaires each related to one of the four patient dependency categories and a general ward based questionnaire. As with the Rush-Medicus System patients are allocated a questionnaire according to their dependency group. The authors recommend that either a random sample of three patients per dependency category are selected or the whole ward be included. Each questionnaire is divided into four sections:
- Assessment of nursing care.
- Meeting the patient's physical needs.
- The patient's non-physical needs are met.
- Evaluation of nursing care objectives.

Sources of information for the question answers include direct patient questioning/observation, patient's records/charts, observation of the clinical environment and questioning of nursing staff.

Answers to questions are scored (Table 3) and a final score is obtained by deducting the non-applicable responses and then dividing the total score by the number of applicable questions and expressing this as a percentage. The authors suggest a score of 70 per cent is desirable. It is recommended that Monitor be carried out in wards once a year.

Answer	
Yes, Yes always, Yes complete	= 1
Yes sometimes, Yes incomplete	= ½
No	= 0

Table 3. Scoring Method For Monitor.

Monitor has been criticised for suggesting a desirable score. Many feel it is better to allow individual ward sisters and nurse managers to decide what is appropriate for their units. For many, a score of less than 100 per cent on knowledge of cardiac arrest procedure or fire drill is unacceptable, while a temporary lapse in other areas, eg evaluating nursing care objectives may be acceptable in a given set of circumstances, such as high vacancy factor/high proportion of new appointees. It has also been criticised for its method of selecting a patient sample, which differs considerably from the Rush-Medicus System of randomly selecting 10 per cent of the patient monthly turnover, irrespective of their dependency groups. Administration is time consuming, particularly in the scoring of the questionnaires, which if done manually can take one person about two working days to complete.

In its favour it must be said that Monitor is a quality monitoring tool developed by a British team who understand the NHS and nursing in the UK and while it is easy to criticise with hindsight, at least North West Region did more than just talk about quality assurance. Monitor has now been adopted by several health authorities in Britain which enjoy a support and update service from Suppliers, Newcastle Polytechnic.

Which programme

Quality Assurance is here to stay, of that there can be little doubt. Hospitals considering implementing a quality assurance programme have two distinct choices; they can either create their own in-house programme or adopt a programme that is commercially available. There are advantages to both. In-house programmes can produce a high level of commitment, creativity and cohesion; bought-in programmes avoid the exercise of reinventing the wheel and have an easily identified price tag and running costs with no hidden extras. Whatever method is chosen by nursing managements it must accurately reflect and measure the quality of care delivered to the patients within the relevant clinical areas.

References

Goldstone, L.A. Ball, J.A. Collier M.M. (1984). MONITOR – An Index of the Quality of Nursing Care for Acute Medical and Surgical Wards. (2nd Impression). Newcastle Upon Tyne Polytechnic Products UK.

Pearson, A. (1983). The Clinical Nursing Unit. (1st Edition). Heinemann Medical Books Ltd, London.

Phaneuf, M. (1976). The Nursing Audit. Appleton-Century-Crofts. New York. USA.

Wandelt, M. and Ager, J. (1974). Quality Patient CAre Scale (QUALPACS). Appleton-Century-Crofts. New York. USA.

Bibliography

Burford Nursing Development Unit. A Compendium of Articles Published in British Nursing Journals by Staff at BNDU (1983–84). (Available on application to BNDU Burford, Oxfordshire).

27

Objectives for care: replacing procedures with guidelines

Gillian Snowley, M.Ed, BSc, RGN, DN
District Education Manager, Mid-Trent College of Nursing and Midwifery

Peter J. Nicklin, M.Ed, RGN, RMN, RNT
Director of Nurse Education, York Health Authority

Since the inception of the NHS, demands upon the service and its employees have increased. Medical technology, demographic change, consumer expectation and managerial concerns for improved productivity, have all conspired to increase the workload of the caring professions. As these demands have intensified, there has been a tendency to forget the importance of the consumer's identity and personal needs. The nursing profession has recognised and acknowledged this neglect, and attempted to provide a solution by adopting the nursing process as a broad philosophy for the planning and delivery of healthcare.

Definitions of the 'nursing process' vary, but common to all are the assumptions that it is goal-directed, systematic, rational and problem-solving. The registered nurse is accountable for delivery of care, based on an assessment of the individual's needs, and for subsequent measurement of the effectiveness (evaluation) of that care. Implementing the nursing process continues to pose significant problems for the profession. The Nurse Education Research Unit (1986) has provided valuable insights into the difficulties experienced by nurses.

A significant barrier

In 1983, the North Lincolnshire Health Authority acknowledged that the 'nursing procedure manual' was a significant barrier to the successful implementation of the nursing process, as it gave no scope for an individualised and prescriptive approach to care. With its rampant and unbending concentration on task, the perfect completion of which would follow the same format on every occasion, the patient's individual needs seemed insignificant. All patients were expected to respond equally, and all nurses to behave with almost military precision on every occasion, despite any special circumstances which could prevail. The procedure manual restricted professional clinical freedom and became a recipe book for nursing. It also encouraged disregard for the psychosocial aspects of care delivery.

This was not to say that procedures were inaccurate, or that accuracy in performing procedures was and is unimportant or unnecessary. But they omitted extra dimensions of care which allow total consideration of the patient. The procedure manual tended to dictate specific technical and highly visible nursing actions in a ritualistic manner, with no concern for assessment, planning and evaluation of nursing care. It did not recognise the individual nurse's role in the process of care delivery – except perhaps for the favourite opening instruction: "Tell the patient what you are going to do". Even that became a regulation!

In 1983, North Lincolnshire's chief nursing officer recommended that "guidelines for nursing practice, which reflect acceptable standards of care" be formulated. Membership of the nursing guidelines committee was drawn from all the health units within the district, including the nurse education unit, so all nurses, midwives and health visitors were represented. The authors were members of this group.

Conceptual differences

During the early stages, we experienced some difficulty in grasping the conceptual differences between 'procedure' and 'guideline', and had little idea what the latter would look like. The prospect of reinventing the wheel did not inspire much enthusiasm, so we undertook the obligatory literature search to determine what had been published in this area. There was little or no information from UK sources, but American literature, while describing a guidelines approach, did not seem to offer anything very different, and was not always consistent with Lincolnshire nursing culture. However, we acknowledged that what we were calling 'guidelines' may not have been so defined by the rest of the nursing profession. Informal discussions with colleagues both regionally and nationally did not reveal any formal work of a similar nature, although it may well have existed. Work subsequently published by the Royal Marsden Hospital (Pritchard and David, 1988) while sharing some of the characteristics of our guidelines, was not entirely consistent with our philosophy. This meant we could not rely on precedents for guidance, but we were not going to distort someone else's structure to fit our own circumstances. In short, we started from scratch.

Although we did not realise it for some time, we needed to ask the question "what does nursing seek to achieve?" Certainly the procedure manual does not answer this. Once we had recognised the importance of the question, we needed to examine models of nursing to identify the structure of nursing guidelines. We considered Orem's (self-care), Roper et al's (activities of living) and Roy's (adaptation model), but eventually returned to basics – to Virginia Henderson's Basic Principles of Nursing Care (1969), which fulfilled our need for a comprehensive and readily understood model. The committee then began composing guidelines under the headings originally described by Henderson.

To say this was difficult would be an understatement. Our first attempts were either too long, too short, too esoteric, too academic, too trivial, too general or too detailed – and sometimes several of these combined! We had problems with semantics and grammar, and our morale sometimes slumped, but by a process of trial and error, consultation and cooperation, we agreed a style of describing nursing intention which had the potential for improving patient care.

Early guidelines

Our early guidelines were expressed as the aims and objectives of nursing on psychosocial, physiological and educational dimensions. Each had an evaluation component, but their most important feature was that each was generated from available literature and published research, and supported by a bibliography.

By late 1985, the committee had developed and disseminated 17 guidelines to all care points in the district. In addition to Henderson's 14 components of basic nursing care, we acknowledged the need to provide guidance on expressing sexuality; helping patients in pain and the care of the dying and bereaved.

Guidelines were intended to be used by trained nurses who can responsibly and reasonably interpret them with discretion and with the authority which the research base provides. We believed they should encourage thoughtful and individual delivery of care by nurses who are accountable for their own actions. The guidelines were recognised as the basis for teaching nurses in training, and for the use of nursing assistants with trained supervision.

Mixed reception

Not surprisingly, our guidelines had a mixed reception in the clinical areas where they were intended to be used. Their appearance coincided with many other recent changes in the philosophy and implementation of healthcare delivery, both nationally and locally directed. Many nurses regarded them as "just another new idea thrust upon us by nurse managers and nurse educators" – despite the fact that clinical nurses from all specialties were members of the committee, and joint authors of the guidelines. One specific problem was that they were seen as isolated documents, and not as an integral part of a systematic and prescriptive approach to individual care. Suddenly, the procedure manual became a highly valued lifeline, even though in many areas it gathered dust and its whereabouts remained unknown. In considering this dilemma, the committee suggested that guidelines were an important aid to the implementation of the nursing process, and that every opportunity to present them as such be pursued. The Open University's Distance Learning Course P553 – A Systematic Approach to Nursing Care (1984) was widely used within the district, both in the continuing education department and within individual units, where courses were being led by nurse managers. The guidelines were therefore introduced to staff undertaking this course as a tool for goal setting and care planning within whichever nursing model was being used in the clinical area. In fact, they provided suitably phrased goals and objectives which would not disgrace any care plan. Although the committee members recognised a responsibility for ensuring such progress and integration of materials, the real work, on a large scale, was done by clinical nurses themselves, with encouragement and facilitation by management and education.

Despite the suspicion and antagonism with which guidelines were received, enough clinical nurses suggested ways in which they could be improved. Members of the committee were grateful for this information – at least in some areas they had not been ignored. Strong statements of dissatisfaction, accompanied by notes of guidance for change, were far more acceptable than apathy.

Revising the format

Armed with suggestions for a changed format, the committee began the formidable task of revision in 1986. This was almost more difficult than beginning with a blank sheet. The original philosophy remained intact, but presentation of the guidelines now evolved into a staged format of assessment, planning, implementation and evaluation. The original objectives, sometimes the results of agonising search for the right expression, remained; so too did the bibliographies, but each has been updated and refined. The result is Objectives for Care, a source book for all nurses, midwives and health visitors, working in any practice setting. This book is the product of an energetic group who were convinced at the outset of the value of the task which confronted them. Some of us had little idea of its enormity, but the team effort involved was its most encouraging aspect.

The book has now been published and every care point in the district has received a copy to replace the old guidelines folder. No doubt it will attract some criticism, as well as some degree of welcome. We sincerely hope it will not remain out of sight long enough to attract dust!

● *Objectives for Care is available from Wolfe Publishing, 2–16 Torrington Place, London.*

References

Henderson, V. (1969) *Basic Principles of Nursing Care*. ICN, Geneva.
NERU (1986) *Report of the Nursing Process Working Party*. King's College, London.
Open University (1984) *A Systematic Approach to Nursing Care – An Introduction* (P553). OU Press, Milton Keynes.
Pritchard, A.P. and David J. (1988) *The Royal Marsden Hospital Manual of Clinical Nursing Policies and Procedures*. Harper and Row, London.

28

Appraisal methods: how do you rate yourself?

Elizabeth S. Wright, SRN, DipN, CHSM
Senior Nurse, Surgical Unit, The Royal London Hospital, Whitechapel, London

Attitudes towards appraisal

A formal system of appraisal is necessary, but which method is most effective? If the whole tactic of appraisal is altered with an aim to improve staff development and career prospects, rather than concentrating solely on criticism of current performance, then the procedure appears much more worthwhile, with long-term planning and objectives designed for the individual's progress, either for her present job or for a different or more senior post.

In the majority of cases within the nursing profession, appraisals are irregular and often serve no constructive purpose for the appraisee. The existence of a staff appraisal interview system compels supervisors to meet with their staff and consult with them on a regular basis, and hence become better informed as to their interests and aspirations (Ansty, 1961). It is insufficient for junior staff nurses to have annual appraisals if they only remain in a junior post for 6 months to a year, and more frequent discussion is necessary to evaluate their progress and needs.

In many professions, including nursing, managers seem reluctant to make any assessment or constructive criticism of their staff. They either avoid doing appraisals or provide ineffective criticisms because they fear to point out weaknesses in performance. This may reflect their inexperience and lack of instruction in methods of appraisal, or possibly their awareness of how difficult it is to make just and accurate assessments, combined with a fear of hostile reactions on confrontation with the appraisee (Fletcher, 1985).

Professional conduct

Being an assessor is a difficult position in which to find yourself, particularly if you work closely with the individual concerned; for instance a sister and a staff nurse working on the same ward. My personal feeling is that one's professional conduct as a senior and therefore a manager, should provide a role model for the staff nurse. The relationship should be friendly and one of approachability and respect, but not familiarity, otherwise the position of assessor loses the credibility necessary for objective criticism to be made. It is to be hoped that the advice will then be received as serious and constructive, and acted upon with intent to improve performance. Managers might find the act of appraisal difficult precisely because they have not maintained a professional relationship with their junior staff.

Current appraisal methods

The most important criterion for a successful method of appraisal is that the manager actually knows the individual concerned, and more importantly her work. Otherwise how can the criticism, good or bad, be justified? How well thought out and personal is the method of appraisal where one person writes a report and another presents it to the individual (commonly a student nurse), often without discussion?

It is preferable that the appraisal is based on first-hand information, but this should include assessment of performance over a substantial period of time, not biased by recent incidents. An overall view of merit is taken into account and should not be marred by personal prejudice.

A common standard by which to assess is difficult to maintain; but in general one should try not to compare to others in a similar post. Assess a person on their own merits in comparison to the standard and experience they should have expected to have attained by that position and after that length of time in the post (Ansty, 1961).

Staff development and career planning

The appraisal may be considered by some managers, and even appraisees, to be an unnecessarily time-consuming process that does not appear to give immediate practical results. An appraisal also involves committing convictions and opinions to paper, which the nurse manager may wish to avoid especially if challenged by the appraisee.

The professional development has long-term implications for clinical practice, but it is not sufficient for the nurse manager to make these assessments and the consequent decisions alone. In order for the most benefit to be gained from the system it is essential that the appraisee is involved in making decisions jointly with the assessor (Pincus, 1982).

I am sure that the fundamental criteria on which to undertake an appraisal, are familiar to all, but they should nevertheless be maintained; such as ensuring a quiet, undisturbed, informal setting, with adequate time set aside. The appraisal needs to be a joint participative exercise between the nurse and her immediate manager in an ambience that is conducive to open discussion, and with strict confidentiality (Stewart, 1978).

The format of the written appraisal form varies greatly between Health Authorities, and the complexity of it depends upon the grade of staff. The actual written evidence of the appraisal is not as important as the two-way discussion. However, it should be completed for reasons of referral and possibly written references at a later date, and as confirmation that the appraisal took place.

Self-appraisal

An increasingly popular and effective method of appraisal which has been implemented in Bloomsbury is self-assessment or self-appraisal. Essentially, the appraisees consider their own ability and skills, and fills out their own appraisal form. The principal advantage of this system is that the appraisees have more opportunity than anyone else to note their own performance and understand their own opinions and conscience, related to weaknesses and strengths within that performance. Self-appraisees are also unlikely to become defensive in response to their own critical analysis of their abilities, although this may prove a natural reaction to another person's criticism. Experience shows that appraisees are more willing to act upon weaknesses or problems that they themselves have identified (Fletcher, 1985).

Although the staff nurse fills out her own appraisal form, it is imperative that her manager discusses each description with her, in order to give an outsider's point of view and assist the nurse's insight with guidance on how to make improvements in each area.

Appraisees seem to be modest in their ratings and realistically a manager needs to guide and help develop the appraisee's skills in self-assessment. The manager may assist in improving not only various practical skills, but also the appraisee's insight into areas of professional development. More importantly, the manager can take the opportunity to give the appraisee credit and praise for work and skills completed with thoroughness and initiative.

How do we meet the many needs of newly qualified staff

A Professional Development Course designed for newly qualified staff nurses is being implemented in Bloomsbury, London. Self-appraisal is incorporated into this course, and is particularly relevant to newly qualified staff who have yet to develop fully the skills of a trained nurse and manager and who require considerable guidance and support in their new role. The project is being undertaken in response to the recognised need for nurses' development in both clinical and professional aspects in the newly qualified staff nurse role, as discussed at the national conference on "Professional Developments in Clinical Nursing – The 1980s", which took place in Harrogate in 1981.

It is the belief of those participating in the professional development course that self-appraisal by the course participants is more appropriate than assessment by examination, because the act of self-appraisal and the personal involvement in setting new targets for achievement serves to take the individual further in their personal development.

Emphasis is therefore placed on self-assessment with related discussion. The format used ultimately provides a detailed descriptive profile of the nurses' strengths and weaknesses in relation to the course objectives, and outlines developmental progress by a comparison of pre-course and post-course assessment profiles. The course members' self-assessment is supplemented by their facilitator's and tutors' comments on their progress.

The course has a six-month programme consisting of supervised and supported practice in a designated training area, involving a facilitator for guidance and practical advice (often the ward sister). The course aims to provide the nurses with the necessary background, awareness, and motivation to pursue a continuous programme of personal development, both clinical and professional. It enables them to develop leadership skills, and prepares them to function as responsible members of the profession. The outline of the course comprises two parts: part one consists of practice under supervision, with emphasis on the clinical role of the registered nurse with a problem-solving context; and part two aims at individual development, which incorporates writing skills, teaching methods, research, and career development as well as leadership skills, within a team and as a practising clinician. Other subjects involving some theoretical tuition are models of nursing and legal and ethical aspects of nursing. The final three study days of the course include seminar presentations by the participants, based on assignment work done during the course, and a concluding debate on professional issues (Smythe, 1984).

I have been facilitator for newly qualified staff nurses who have completed the six-month course. The course has been beneficial to them in providing theoretical support for practical issues and practice. It has encouraged them to seek further education and develop their careers with a confident and inquiring insight into the practice carried out on the wards. The course also allowed me to evaluate the support and needs I was trying to fulfil for my staff nurses. Perhaps other ward sisters should do likewise?

As previously mentioned, this course commenced as a pilot scheme and it was not intended for general implementation until the advantages and disadvantages have been fully assessed and evaluated after 3 years.

I believe that much of the negative feelings that I have expressed regarding staff appraisal result from the fact that so many managers are not taught proper methods of appraisal, and often carry it out ineffectively. There has to be a better way, and I am sure that self-appraisal incorporated into a professional development scheme is a more positive and effective method of identifying the individuals' needs, and of improving and praising their abilities.

References

Anstey, E., (1971) Staff Reporting and Development. George Allen & Unwin Ltd., London.
Fletcher, C., (1985) Means of assessment. *Nursing Times*, **81;27,**24
Filkins, J., (1985) Going round in circles. *Nursing Times*, **81;29,**31
Pincus, J., (1982) Staff appraisal and development. *Nursing Mirror*, **155;21,**47
Smythe, J. E., (1984) Professional development of the newly registered nurse; Guidelines in the Bloomsbury scheme. Unpublished.
Stewart, A. M., (1978) Staff development and peformance review. *Nursing Times*, **74;16,**654.

Bibliography
Dimmock, S., (1985) Starting from scratch. *Nursing Times*, 81;30.
Jessup, G., and Jessup, H., (1975) Selection and Assessment at Work. Methuen & Co. Ltd., London.
Randell, G., Shaw, R., Packard, P., Slater, J. (1972) Staff Appraisal. Institute of Personnel Management, London.
Raybould, E., (1977) Editor. Guide for Nurse Managers. Blackwell Scientific Publications, London.

29

How well do we perform? Parents' perceptions of paediatric care

Margaret Ball, BN, RGN
Teaching Assistant, Department of Nursing Studies

Alan Glasper, BA, RGN, RSCN, ONC, DN, CertEd, RNT
Professor of Nursing Studies

Paul Yerrell, BSc, PhD
Visiting Fellow, Department of Nursing Studies, all at the University of Southampton

Towards the end of 1987, staff on the Paediatric Unit at Southampton General Hospital were worried by staff shortages and associated low morale. There were fears that standards of care could be falling, so there developed a keen interest to measure the quality of care on the unit.

Quality is defined by Roberts (1975) as a grade of goodness, ie it is a measurement. Quality assurance is a process of looking at a given situation and appraising it against a measure or a set standard. In the nursing context this enables nurses to promise and maintain a set standard of care. Setting standards is a vital part in this process which the RCN is pursuing with its standards of care project (Kitson, 1988).

Assessing quality of care

One of the most frequently used frameworks for looking at quality of care is that developed by Donabedian (1976). This is based on three distinct, but interrelated factors; structure, process and outcome. Structure looks at the environmental and resource items and their organisation. Process refers to the planning and delivery of the nursing interventions and outcome is concerned with the result of care. Kitson (1988) has devised a model which can be used to look at these three aspects. She describes the process of quality assurance as cyclic, consisting of describing the problem, measuring it and then taking action. Each of these areas can then be broken down into more specific steps (Figure 1). As the process is cyclic it can be entered at any point.

Quality assurance is a subject very much in vogue. Many tools have been developed, such as Monitor, which has been adapted from an American version by Goldstone (1983). Some of these are being used in the clinical setting to evaluate and measure quality of care. In America,

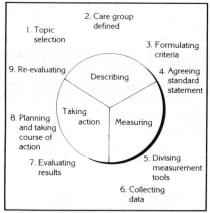

Figure 1. The process of quality assurance.

quality assurance programmes are much more developed than ours, partly because of their private health care system, in which insurance companies demand to know standards of care, but also because of their higher levels of medical litigation. In the UK there has been an increasing recognition of the need for work on quality, which has developed for numerous reasons. Of particular influence has been the implementation of Griffiths style management with its emphasis on cost effectiveness. Also, the public are becoming more medically aware, and their expectations of the health services are increasing.

Quality assurance in paediatrics

Little work has been done on quality assurance in the paediatric field. Some previous work by Maddison (1977) highlighted the importance of seeking the opinion of consumers. Maddison believes parental opinion is most valid in paediatrics in that it reflects that of the child. She further states that she would like to see a grading system for evaluating paediatric wards similar to the stars used to grade hotels. This grade would be strongly influenced by the degree of emotional support offered to children and their parents.

Brykczynska (1987) points out that nurses must work with the child and family, not against them or in spite of them. The child should be viewed as a partner in care, and further work to ascertain children's perceptions of their own care be undertaken.

For the purposes of this pilot study in addressing the staff's worries about care, it was decided to ascertain parental views on the quality of their children's nursing care. This was seen as a way of identifying problems upon which standards of care may be set and further quality work carried out. Although parental opinion is one way of measuring quality of care, it has limitations, because parents' perceptions only relate to perceived quality of care. These do not take into account actual outcome or necessarily reflect the standards of the nursing staff.

The tool chosen to do this was a questionnaire based on some work done at the Hospital for Sick Children in Toronto. It consists of some open-ended questions and some forced choice Likert scale questions in which parents are asked to strongly agree, agree, disagree or strongly disagree to numerous statements (Figure 2). The questionnaire looks at many areas of paediatric nursing care and covers aspects of structure, process and outcome.

A recent article by Ledwith (1988) notes the recent popularity of

For the following statements please check the response which most closely reflects your opinion.	1 Strongly Disagree	2 Disagree	3 Agree	4 Strongly Agree
1. I received consistent information/instructions from each nurse caring for my child during the hospital stay.				
2. I was given adequate information about my child's ward.				
3. I received no information about hospital rules and procedures that might have applied to my family and me.				
4. The nurses always responded to my requests promptly.				
5. The nurses and I discussed how my child's illness or hospitalisation would affect me and my family.				
6. The nurses always asked if I understood what the doctor told me.				
7. I always had trouble getting a nurse when I needed one.				
8. The nurses asked me what I would like to know about my child's illness or hospitalisation.				
9. I feel confident in the nurses caring for my child.				
10. The nurses protected my child's privacy.				
11. I feel confident that I can manage my child's care at home after discharge.				
12. All the nurses caring for my child were familiar with the care he/she needed.				
13. The nurses fully involved me in the planning of my child's nursing care and in the writing of the care plan.				
14. I had to answer a lot of the same questions about my child's needs many times.				
15. If my child was fearful or anxious during any procedures the nurse attempted to reassure, comfort and calm him/her.				
16. I feel the nurses would be willing to stay with my child if he/she was worried or upset about something.				
17. The nurses talked with me and my family about what we could expect to happen during my child's hospitalisation.				
18. I received adequate information about tests and procedures from my child's nurses.				
19. My child received explanation from the nurse that he/she could understand before any procedure was started.				
20. The nurses never asked me how I would prefer my child's care to be carried out.				
21. The nurses helped me feel comfortable in participating in my child's care.				
22. The nurses attended to my child's likes and dislikes as best they could.				
23. The nurses showed genuine interest and concern for my child.				
24. I felt comfortable asking the nurses any questions.				

25. Did you stay with your child during the hospital admission? YES/NO If Yes, was it?: a) on the ward b) in a cubicle c) in Victoria House?
26. What in your opinion was most helpful to you during the period of time your child was in hospital? Please comment:
27. What could have made the hospital stay better for you as a parent/guardian? Please comment:
28. How would you rate your child's nursing care on this ward. A Excellent C Fair B Good D Poor
29. Date today ....
Your additional comments would be most welcome. Thank you.

Figure 2. The questionaire (adapted with kind permission of the Hospital for Sick Children, Toronto).

consumer surveys in the NHS but emphasises that these should look at the quality of information and support, not just overall patient satisfaction. A single criteria to measure quality may be suited to commercial organisations, but is not sufficient in health care. Work on interpersonal communication has shown communication processes and information levels in the health service have a direct effect on consumer satisfaction. The questionnaire was designed to explore these areas.

The effect of staff-client relationships

Barbarin and Chesler (1984) commented that in areas where staff-client relationships are good, quality of care was better than in those where interpersonal relationships were poor. Their study found respect for medical staff strongly related to parents' perceptions of the transmission of information and their evaluation of the staff's technical competence. Francis et al (1969) found mothers were more likely to comply with treatment when staff were understanding, warm and friendly.

Sheridan (1975) has pointed out that children honour those people who tell the truth about procedures, especially where pain is involved. Good communication helps to minimise the disturbance caused by hospital admission. Other work has found parents of hospitalised children to be highly motivated learners (Aufhauser and Lesh, 1973) who then take information to the community where it is most needed.

The questionnaire was administered to the parents of the first 10 children discharged from each of four paediatric wards in the last week of January 1988. Ward clerks were felt to be the best people to administer them, being the most neutral people on the wards with no direct care input. Complete anonymity was guaranteed and the final sample number was 35; five questionnaires were incompletely answered or not returned.

Results of the survey

Overall the results of the questionnaire demonstrated that parents were satisfied with the care they and their children received. Despite the inherent 'halo' effect commonly seen with this type of research, much valuable data was obtained. Only 8.1 per cent described their child's care as fair, while the remaining 91.4 per cent described it as excellent or good (60 per cent excellent; 31.4 per cent good).

Parents particularly liked being able to stay with their children in hospital and 75.9 per cent of the sample were resident during their child's admission. Written comments revealed that parents greatly appreciated the relaxed atmosphere found on the wards, and many were delighted with the play facilities on offer. All respondents felt they could manage their child's care at home following discharge.

The results did highlight some areas of care where parents were not fully satisfied. Several questions were specifically targeted at information-giving, and the results show there is a need for more information to be given to parents; 33.4 per cent indicated that nursing staff did not ask them if they understood what the doctor had told them and a small number said they did not receive adequate information about the ward or about tests and procedures (11.4 per cent). Some parents (8.6 per cent) felt that information given to them was not always consistent and a minority (5.7 per cent) did not feel comfortable asking nurses questions. Several comments in response to the 'open-ended' questions also reflected this need for more information for parents.

The impact of hospitalisation

The impact of hospitalisation on children and families was addressed in several questions. Responses show this is an area where parents are critical: 38.2 per cent felt there was insufficient discussion by nurses on the effect hospitalisation might have on themselves and their families, and a quarter (25.7 per cent) indicated that nurses did not talk to them about what would happen to their children in hospital.

Parents were highly complimentary about their children's nursing care and attitudes among staff. There were some areas, however, where parental expectations were not met: 40 per cent reported that nurses did not involve them in planning care and a similar number reported that nurses never asked them how they would like their child's care to be carried out. The concept of parental involvement in the care of sick children was also highlighted by several comments indicating that parents would like to do more for their children. Two parents specifically reported that the nursing staff did not make them feel comfortable in participating in their child's care while 14.3 per cent believed that some nurses were not familiar with the care their children needed.

A small number of parents reported that nurses did not respond promptly to requests, but believed this was mitigated by the pressure of work. Several commented on the ward environment; some noted that toys and furniture were not very clean. Comments were also received on excessive noise, such as squeaky doors, and such irritations were thought to be controllable. Some parents were concerned about lighting levels. Some said the lights were too bright at night and suggested darker curtains between cubicles, while others felt greater segregation of children into age groups would allow lights to be turned off earlier for younger children.

A few parents wanted to eat with their children and were reluctant to go to the canteen, calling for more eating facilities on the ward. It is interesting that some parents said they wanted tea and coffee facilities when these facilities did exist on all wards.

In conclusion, the majority of parents identified care to be of a good or excellent standard. In respect to information, hospitalisation, parental involvement, and facilities for parents, a minority of parents saw room for improvements. Here we are reminded of Ledwith's reservation that although overall satisfaction is a useful measure, it is not sufficient in the health service.

Addressing parents' concerns

In the interests of the children we care for, we may need to address the concerns highlighted in this work within the financial and manpower constraints imposed upon clinical areas. With regard to information giving, the results encourage nurses to give parents more information both formally and informally. New areas being explored are preadmission programme, a care by parent scheme, ward booklets and discharge information packs. Nurses are also encouraged to examine how to involve parents more fully in their child's care. The advantages of care by parent schemes such as that initiated in Cardiff (Sainsbury et al, 1986) may result in their continued growth and development in the UK.

While responses to the questionnaire indicate areas where nurses could improve care, the task still remains to describe the structure, process and outcome criteria which will allow specific standards to be set, against which a measurement of quality can be made. Restraints of time may well be hindering nurses in this task and perhaps the results of this pilot study will raise awareness and prompt nurses to look at the issues involved.

We should remind ourselves that if we are to promote nursing as a research-based profession, we should be using the plethora of nursing research to help us achieve our goals of identifying problems, setting standards and measuring quality of care. It will be, of course, for each paediatric unit, as they embark on setting standards in relation to the quality of care, to decide what proportion of time they devote to setting and measuring standards in relation to problems evolving from parents' perceptions. Only when practitioners identify a personal commitment to changing practice and recognise the role parents' views might have in identifying where changes are required, will paediatric units become fully self-evaluating.

References

Aufhauser, T.R. and Lesh, D. (1973) Parents need TLC too. *Hospital*, **47**, 8,88.
Barbarin, O. and Chesler, M.A. (1984) Relationships with the medical staff and aspects of satisfaction with care expressed by parents of children with cancer. *Journal of Community Health*, **9**, 4, 302–13.
Brykczynska, G.M. (1987) Ethical issues in paediatric nursing. *Nursing*, **3**, 2, 862–864.
Donabedian, A. (1976) Measures of quality of care. *American Journal of Nursing*, **76**, 2, 186.
Francis, V. et al (1969) Gaps in doctor – patient communication response to medical advice. *New England Journal of Medicine*, **280**, 535–540.
Goldstone, L.A. et al (1983) Monitor. Newcastle upon Tyne Polytechnic Products Limited.
Kitson, A.L. (1988) Nursing Quality Assurance. Dynamic Standard Setting System. RCN Standards of Care Project, unpublished.
Ledwith, F. (1988) Doing less to achieve more. *Health Service Journal*, **98**, 3088.
Maddison, M. (1977) Consumer survey of paediatric wards. *Australian Nurses' Journal*, **6**, 1, 27–28.
Roberts, I. (1975) Discharged from hospital. Royal College of Nursing, London.

Sainsbury, C.P.Q. et al (1986) Care by parents of their children in hospital. *Archives of Disease in Childhood*, **61**, 612–615.
Sheridan, M.S. (1975) Children's feelings about the hospital. *Social Work in Health Care*, **1**, 65–70.

30

Self-evaluation can protect your competence

Patrick McEvoy, RMN, SRN, DipN(Lond), RCNT, RNT, BA
Senior Tutor, Department of Post Basic Education, Easton Area College of Nursing Southside

Who really knows the truth about us but ourselves? Even our professional lives can be a closed book to all but our internal censor. This is why self-evaluation is crucial for professional development. As health professionals nurses, of course, are subjected to formal evaluation at virtually every turn and corner of their careers, which begins during interviews for courses and jobs. It is the primary purpose of examinations and assessments, whether they are formative or summative. Although much stress is placed on the developmental aspect of periodic staff review, appraisal is an all too obvious aspect of the proceedings. Even organisational meetings are sometimes used to evaluate the performance of individuals. Then there are those managers who will remark glibly, 'Call up and see me some time', usually with none of the connotations reminiscent of Mae West. Their covert intention is informal counselling, which can be a polite precurser of a formal warning. Performance indicators and value-for-money scrutinies are recent additions to the arsenal of evaluation which afflicts professionals within the health service.

Measuring quality

Following the Griffiths Report in 1983, an upsurge of interest in the optimal use of limited resources spawned a renewed application of quality assurance methods which had been emanating from the United States since 1980. Techniques such as Qualpacs and Monitor soon became fashionable as measures of quality. These rather obtuse instruments merely measure standards of care within broad parameters. Terms like 'average care', 'above average care', 'best nurse' and 'poorest nurse' do little to inspire the individual practitioner towards excellence in professional practice.

"To use Qualpacs, nurses must clarify their own value systems and identify their own standards," wrote Barnett and Wainwright (1987). This can only be done through enlightened self-evaluation. "Audit/evaluative methods such as Qualpacs measure quality, but these methods alone can only marginally improve quality. There is only one way to substantially improve quality. Every employee in the organisation needs to accept and understand that quality starts and ends with him," said Ryland and Richards (1987). In other words, only self-evaluation will assure quality of care.

By its very nature, formal evaluation is quantitative rather than qualitative. It is concerned with percentages, grades and measurable results. It produces faithful recording of the nursing process regardless of actual standards of care. It ensures that tutors amass lesson plans, remain in class for the full 60 minutes, and show a presence on the wards without indicating anything of the quality of their teaching. At best, formal evaluation can only enforce minimum standards. It seldom inspires excellence. Regardless of all the interviews, examinations, appraisals and even formal warnings, the real race for excellence is the one you run against yourself.

The reflective practitioner

Self-evaluation is the hallmark of the reflective practitioner. Indeed, it is the hallmark of the mature person in any walk of life. It is a vital ingredient of the hidden curriculum which interlaces every interaction between client and professional. It is all about creating and measuring excellence within professional functions and relationships. Essentially, it involves asking, 'What have I to offer these (patients) (students) (clients) that they are unlikely to get from any other source?' I asked myself this question repeatedly as I penned this article; and my answer has been, "A series of ideas, beliefs, reflections and bits of humour, hopefully linked together in such a way as to inspire the reader to ask some pertinent questions of himself." Perhaps you would like to begin by answering the following questions:

1. I frequently/sometimes/seldom take time out to reflect on my own professional performance.
2. I frequently/sometimes/seldom read stimulating literature which is related to my work.
3. I frequently/sometimes/seldom seek verbal and nonverbal cues from the recipients of my professional endeavours which will assist my efforts at self-evaluation.
4. I frequently/sometimes/seldom feel that I am gaining professional self-confidence as I grow older.
5. I frequently/sometimes/seldom ask myself, "If I were the purchaser of my own services would I be satisfied with what I am providing?"
6. I frequently/sometimes/seldom feel that I am governed by 'the tyranny of the urgent'.

The last question is the odd one out. While it is desirable that you can answer 'frequently' to the others, it is ideal if you are seldom governed by 'the tyranny of the urgent'. Do you often moan that you have not the time to read professional literature because you are too busy? Is your desk cluttered? Do you always seem to be working under pressure? Worse still, are you a victim of adhocracy or institutional disorganisation? These can blight your professional life. The reflective practitioner will avoid taking on more than he or she can accomplish calmly and effectively. Time, like money, must be budgeted. If nurses were as careful with time as they tend to be with money, their professional effectiveness barometer would take a meteoric rise.

Self-esteem

Self-evaluation is closely related to self-esteem. Self-esteem is the evaluation which an individual makes of his personal worth, competence and significance. Maxwell Maltz (1968) claims that 95 per cent of people feel inferior. He does not say how much of the time or to what degree. Low professional self-esteem may be due to past failures: for example, failure to win a cherished promotion, or a bad experience while teaching in the classroom. Interstaff relationships may also be damaging. There are always those who attempt to boost their own self-esteem at someone else's expense. The astute professional will avoid an inordinate desire to meet other people's expectations. Nor will he feel that he must always be master of his environment. Where people are concerned this is virtually impossible, and will inevitably lead to frustration and feelings of inferiority. This is particularly likely to occur in the clinical setting where staff shortages and expanding needs makes a high degree of control unrealisable.

It may also be perilous to place too much reliance on status symbols to feed one's self-esteem: for example, insistence on the use of titles, letters after one's name, large offices and expensive furnishings. The tutor who insists on being regarded as omnipotent in the classroom has also tied his self-esteem to a status symbol. Such trappings can be superseded through regrading a demand for new qualifications or an emphasis on self-directed learning. Ultimately, retirement will sweep them all away.

Sometimes poor professional self-esteem is a product of the incompetence of others. In a bureaucratic heirarchy people become victims of poor forward planning, lack of communication, unprofessional behaviour, strangulation by red tape and adhocracy. The latter can sometimes be worse than the disease which it attempts to bypass. Reflective self-evaluation can protect a person's self-esteem even within such situations.

Where do we begin with self-evaluation? We must go back over our professional careers and identify those influences that have shaped our present levels of performance. Only when we understand how our present behaviour has developed will we be in a position to evaluate it.

Creating excellence

The reflective professional does not evaluate himself out of mere curiosity, or to compare himself arrogantly with others, or to see how bad he is, but rather to create excellence within himself. For self-evaluation to be effective, we must first develop a concept of the professional we would like to be. This will be personal and subjective; but nonetheless real. Like every other human endeavour, if there is no objective there can be no journey. If we can conceptualise an ideal professional self based upon freely chosen nursing, philosophical, educational and spiritual values, we can continually evaluate ourselves in the light of these. In this way professional self-esteem will be fostered as a personal conviction is developed that the individual is uniquely valuable to the recipients of his or her service, whether patients, clients or students.

Self-evaluation can be a potent source of positive reinforcement. We must try to link self-evaluation with self-reward. What are the rewards and threats which are motivating present behaviour? Self-evaluation linked to self-reward will produce a subtle shift from being externally directed to being internally directed. Individuals who do not learn to reinforce themselves must endlessly seek approval from others. Rewards from others are empty without our own self-regard to back them up.

It is a good idea initially to focus evaluation within our areas of competence. This should result in immediate gratification. As self-esteem is gained, we can move to the less successful aspects of our professional life. For example, we could begin by listing our most satisfying activities, which are most likely to be those that we do well. If self-evaluation shows a consistency in the qualities desired, we can tell ourselves: 'I certainly conducted that meeting smoothly and efficiently'; 'I asserted myself in that situation without damaging anyone's self-esteem'; 'I responded appropriately to that patient who came to me for counselling'.

It is important to be specific in relation to self-reward, and to avoid self-adulation and wishful thinking. The worst of all frauds is to cheat oneself. Share self-evaluation with a trusted colleague, and always remain alert for more objective confirmation of self-judgement. Remember there is often a kernel of truth in all personal criticism, however unfair it may appear at the time.

Journey of self-discovery

Like throwing a pebble into water, the process of self-evaluation continually expands a professional's self-awareness. It is a journey of self-discovery which can make a career more exciting and fruitful. A person evaluating himself can never be completely objective: but then neither will a person appraising another. We all give each other bitter pills to swallow, and we all fall far short of our potential. The success of any method of evaluation must be the extent to which it motivates a person to a more complete development of his talents. Self-evaluation outreaches all other forms of appraisal in that it magnetises a person towards his own centre of excellence.

References
Barnett, D. and Wainwright, P. (1987) Between two tools. *Senior Nurse*, **6**, 4.
Ryland, P. and Richards, F. (1987) Where the buck stops. *Senior Nurse*, **6**, 3.

Bibliography

Bliss, E.C. (1983) Doing it Now. Futura Publications, London.

Hickman, C.R. and Silva, M.A. (1985) Creating Excellence. Allen and Unwin, London.

Kanter, R.M. (1984) The Change Masters. Allen and Unwin, London.

Maltz, M. (1986) Psychocybernetics. Essandes, New York.

Peters, T.J. and Waterman, R.H. (1982) In Search of Excellence. Harper and Row, New York.

Waitley, D. (1984) Seeds of Greatness. Windmill Press, Kingswood, Surrey.

Wayner, M.E. (1975) The Sensation of Being Somebody. Building and adequate self-concept. Zondervan, Grand Rapids.

Financial Resources

31

Managing a budget at ward level

Wanda K. Shafer, RGN, Cert. Man. Studs.
Outpatient Manager, Hillingdon Hospital, Uxbridge

Managing a budget at ward level requires a systematic approach in order to do it well. The essential elements are:
• Good information which is readily available.
• Resource people to provide the much needed support.
• Authority to implement changes.
• A forum which provides evaluation in an ongoing fashion.

Good information

The manager must have a comprehensive knowledge of the current expenditures for the ward.

Computer print-outs of central supplies, stock levels, pharmacy stock levels, inventory of furniture and equipment (asset registry), staff levels and the costs often associated with other departments, i.e., advertising, radiology, theatre, TSSU, etc. These latter costs are often forgotten when budgets are devolved to ward level. Having this information is crucial to the understanding of how the speciality unit/ward relates to the hospital.

Current information regarding staffing levels, skill mix, patient dependency, patterns of workload (i.e., 5-day beds, day cases, ward attenders etc.) is necessary to determine if you are utilising your human resources effectively.

It is extremely important to be aware of any anticipated changes in medical practice which would have an effect on the unit i.e., a purchase of new equipment in theatre or a new minor operation/diagnostic procedure which can be carried out in the outpatient department. These changes can have an affect on the dependency level of the patients on the ward. A change of consultant could have a major knock-on effect which is sometimes not considered in advance.

Nothing can be more important than good communication. Sharing your information, thoughts and asking questions keeps everyone aware of what is happening. It also encourages staff to participate in the problem solving process which strengthens the team and improves the quality of the services you are offering.

Resource people

Central supply   The Radcliffe Infirmary uses a topping up service for those items most frequently used on the ward, i.e., tapes, syringes, needles etc. The level is or can be controlled by the ward.

When I first observed my stores expenditure as a new Senior Sister, I was quite shocked. I wanted it decreased, but I did not want to decrease quality. Initially, I spent what seemed an eternity in "the cupboard", so much time that staff began referring to it as "Sisters office". Once I knew what was on the shelf Mike, the person responsible for topping up, provided a complete list indicating what quantities, when and where they were ordered with a total expenditure for the year.

I spent several hours sorting through this and with Mike's help we set new stock levels. As treatments or needs change, the levels are adjusted. We have also begun to do some "comparison shopping".

Pharmacy   Anyone who has even looked at a ward budget knows that the one area always high in expenditure is Pharmacy. There seems little that can be done. However, you must investigate to ensure there is not high wastage.

We first looked at our ward stock levels, which again, are maintained on a topping-up system by the Pharmacy. It has been my experience that nurses are "be prepared" people. We had stock items which were never touched but were there "just in case". Many times these items would expire and be replaced having never been used. This sort of "shelf wastage", as I refer to it, is very costly.

With the assistance of the pharmacist, and the perseverance of the team leaders, we now have our stock levels in a reasonable state.

Clinical Practice Development Nurses   The highest expenditure in any ward budget is staffing. It is, therefore, always being challenged. The manager must understand and be able to defend her staffing levels. The only way to be able to firmly say your levels are correct is to start at the beginning by developing a ward philosophy, determining how you will organise your nursing (i.e., team nursing, primary nursing, task, patient allocation) and choosing/developing a model of nursing.

Patient dependency: Resource Management Project Nurse   Continuing on from the above, you must now determine what dependency level of patient you have. The Oxford Nurse Management System is based on the work carried out by Dr Sue Pembrey in 1979. It establishes patient need, planned nursing hours, available nursing hours and the cost of nursing care for each patient. The ward staff develop this information utilising their ward philosophy and nursing care plans along with the immense support from the Resource Management Project Nurse. Once this information is available on the computer, it is then possible to look at skill mix to ensure that you have it correct.

Personnel officer   Some of the hidden costs, that can become quite high, have to do with an area of personnel, ie, advertising, annual leave, sick pay, training. It is very important to consult the personnel officer whenever you have a question in these areas.

Medical staff   It cannot be stressed enough that managing a budget at ward level requires team work. Working with the medical staff is imperative and therefore it is up to the ward manager/senior sister to keep communication channels open. This is sometimes a difficult area.

Accountant   A very useful resource person is the accountant, but do keep in mind that they are not always familiar with hospitals, nurses or the fact that there is a human life at issue not a product.

Director of Nursing Services   The Director of Nursing Services is always there and is always needed for consultation, challenge and the ability to offer the personal support to keep you going.

Clinical service manager/Administrative assistant   Whatever your institution may refer to them as, they are indispensable. A non-nursing input that allows you to delegate non-nursing tasks to them. The type of support you need when you are not quite certain who you need to consult – they just seem to always know the answer!

Implementing change

Having all this information and reams of computer print-outs will be of no use if you do not have the authority to implement change. You must be aware at the start what you will have the authority to change and what procedures you must follow. Understanding change and its effect is important for all concerned. Introducing too much too quickly can often produce unwanted results.

Again, keeping all staff informed and involved is essential. Many ideas for change or improvement are initiated by the ward staff. If they are allowed to implement change they will also be willing to accept the responsibility for evaluating the effectiveness of the change.

It is apparent to me, after nearly two years in post, that being ward-based with some clinical involvement is beneficial as it provides the opportunity to see first hand how things are working on the ward and the sorts of issues that arise in the course of the day. Communication channels are also easier to maintain when you are visible.

Evaluating progress

Each specialty unit has a quarterly Management Budgeting meeting. The agenda for this meeting is derived from the accountants financial information pertaining to the specialty. The meeting is chaired by the Unit General Manager and attended by the senior sister, senior consultant, the accountant, the clinical services manager and, if it is a surgical specialty, the theatre manager. This forum allows for reviewing the current situation and highlighting areas that may need extra attention.

In the ENT specialty unit we have determined that extra meetings are needed to address some of our problem areas. We have therefore set up a meeting between the Management Budgeting meetings. We use this forum as an investigative/problem solving meeting and involve members from the multidisciplinary health care team. These have proven useful as we can then report back to the quarterly meeting with our results.

I have only been able to touch on some of the aspects involved in managing a budget at ward level. With each gain that is made, some new areas become apparent which require attention and the whole process begins again.

References
Bagust, A. (1990) Dispel that old myth. *The Health Service Journal,* **6,** 1000–1001.
Brechbiel, K. (1990) Getting a grip on your unit's budget. *American Journal of Nursing,* **90**(1) 42I–42L.
Brechbiel, K. (1990) How to justify your staffing. *American Journal of Nursing,* **9**(5,)28.
Cardin, S. (1990) What's in a (manager's) name? *American Journal of Nursing,* **90**(5)28.
Chalmers, J. (1990) Making resource management work. *Professional Nurse,* **5**(4,)178–80.
Haynes, M. (1987) Make every minute count: How to manage your time effectively. *Crisp Publications,* Los Altos, California.
Williams, S. (1989) The Radcliffe revolution. *Nursing Times,* **85,**18.
Wood, K. (1990) Resource management in action on the ward. *Professional Nurse,* **5**(5,)492–94.

32

Showing where the money goes: cost-effective care in ICU

Karen Ballard, RGN
Sister, ICU, St Peter's Hospital, Chertsey

The nurse practitioner role is centred around delivering the best possible care to patients and their families. The recent proposals outlined in the government's White Paper (DoH, 1989) have raised awareness among nurses that resource management will soon become their responsibility - indeed many ward-based nurses have already taken on the system.

In setting up effective systems of resource management, Griffiths (1983) said each unit must "develop management budgets which involve clinicians and relate workload and service objectives to financial and manpower allocations". A major problem in meeting Griffiths's aim has been that the NHS has no real idea of the individual costs of care. The clinical nurse's role has not been shown to realistically extend to full accountability for the cost of care, and it is vital that whatever changes do occur in the NHS, the quality of care remains paramount. There is little doubt that nurses will become more involved in budgeting care, but valuable nurse manpower must not be misused. Views about nurses' primary role are changing, and a conflict exists between the traditional role of carer at the bedside and the developing role in such areas as resource management. These issues must eventually be solved, and it is up to us as nurses to ensure the solution does not put efficiency and cost-effectiveness above quality of care.

Increasing awareness
In order to prepare for the change to resource management, staff in the intensive care unit (ICU) at St Peter's Hospital, Chertsey decided to find ways of delivering the most cost-effective care without compromising the quality of that care. Many methods can be used to carry out nursing procedures, and these involve diverse pieces of equipment, take variable amounts of time and may result in different levels of effectiveness for the patient. When considering cost-effectiveness, the priority must remain to ensure the patient receives the highest standard of nursing care possible, and our prime consideration had to be that patient safety was in no way compromised. Apart from the potentially devastating effect sub-standard

care could have on our highly dependent patients, savings made at the expense of safety are usually a false economy. Patients may well develop complications as a result of cheaper but poorer quality care, and may cost the NHS more to treat. For example, if pressure relieving aids are not used, particularly with the highly dependent patients in ICU, they may well develop pressure sores, which were estimated to cost the NHS £15,000,000 per year to treat five years ago (Johnson, 1985). Appropriate use of short-acting sedation can be more expensive than longer acting drugs, but can mean the patient requires less time on the ventilator and is highly dependent for less time, making the care cheaper to provide.

Equipment costs

When assessing costs, it is important to consider the amount of nursing time that can be saved when using more expensive items. It is essential that nursing manpower is put to the most appropriate use and this may mean that a more expensive item is indicated. For example, the cost of intravenous infusions with pre added drugs such as potassium or heparin can cost around 40% more than buying the infusion fluid and drugs separately. When you consider the savings in nursing time, the cost of the two methods can be calculated to be roughly the same.

We decided that a good starting point in gaining an awareness of the costs of care would be in concentrating on our use of equipment - of course there are other facets to resource management, such as staffing and skill mix, but we felt equipment costs were an area in which we could all help make savings simply by becoming more aware of the costs of items we used. We began by researching the prices of all items, from the 2.5 pence plastic apron to the £60 pressure monitoring catheter.

Our original assumption that this would be a relatively easy task was far from true - it turned out to be a lengthy process involving staff from stores, pharmacy and the suppliers themselves. Issues to consider included the fact that some companies charge a 25 per cent cancellation fee for standing orders, some prices included VAT or needed a carriage charge to be added, and some companies give discounts for large orders. Eventually, however, we managed to work out reasonably accurate prices for the items we used, and set about displaying them for all to see. Every box, container or cupboard now gives the price of all items it contains, so all the staff - including doctors - can see the cost of the items they use. This alone has generated some interesting conversations about the best choice of equipment for various procedures, and has made staff stop to think before opening items that are not really required.

In finding the prices of equipment, we realised we used many items that could be obtained more cheaply: intravenous (IV) giving sets ranged from 85 pence to £3.70. We could now select the item which gave us the quality we required at the most cost-effective price. The criteria we established for giving sets were: accuracy (20 drops/ml), luer lock connections, whether they needed burettes, and whether they were the appropriate standard. For example, blood giving sets are expensive because they incorporate a filter, which is not necessary when only administering crystalloids.

The quality of urine bags is vital if urinary tract infections are to be minimised by using systems that prevent the reflux of urine. When we looked at the range, we found that cheaper bags were available, but these would have to be changed more frequently, and could be detrimental to patients if they did not give the protection they needed.

Staff awareness

Displaying the prices also made staff more aware of the possible unnecessary wastage caused by poor planning of patient care. For example, some patients will inevitably require multiple infusions, such as inotropes, parenteral feeding and sedation, within 24 hours of the first line being inserted. These patients could have a multiple lumen central line inserted, rather than a single line which would have to be changed for a multiple one within 24 hours, wasting £10.00. Constant reminders of the cost of waste makes all staff more aware of the necessity to plan the care they deliver more effectively.

Care delivery

Having individually priced all the items we use, we began to explore different methods used to deliver care, such as the administration of drug infusions, eye care, bronchial saline lavage and the use of water humidification. Arriving at accurate costings for nursing procedures was extremely difficult, as so many variables require consideration. We took account of factors such as nursing time, the need for more equipment, possible effects on the patient, patient comfort and increased wear and tear on existing equipment, and calculated the most cost-effective methods of carrying out procedures without compromising patient care. It has already been demonstrated (Cousins, 1988) that savings of up to 35 per cent can be made by using the Pall 0.2 micron IV filter, which allows IV disposables to be changed every 96 hours, as opposed to every 24. There are added advantages in that the patient is better protected from microbial and other particulate contamination, endotoxins and air emboli, while nursing time is also saved, and our calculations confirm the figure of 35 per cent savings.

Recent studies (Chalon *et al*, 1984) have shown the Pall heat and moisture exchanging filter in the ventilator circuit acts as an efficient humidifier, and avoids the hazards presented by water humidifiers (Gallagher *et al*, 1987). When we compared the cost of humidification in a ventilated patient using a heat and moisture exchanging filter with installation of saline into the endotracheal tube prior to suction, we calculated that savings of £4,164.65 per bed per year were possible.

Questioning procedures

Although we initially set out to explore the financial aspects of patient care, this involved looking closely at the quality of care being delivered. By questioning our procedures in an effort to be more cost-effective, we were able to improve the quality of patient care. Making the best use of resources in the NHS must be considered by all those working in the services, so patients can receive the best possible care. It has been shown by the studies within our unit that savings can be made without compromising the care we give, but it is essential that where savings are made, budget-holders can use the money saved within their unit, to buy new equipment, fund staff study leave or improve the staff skill mix. This will provide the incentive so desperately needed for staff to make themselves cost-conscious and cost-effective.

References

Chalon, P. et al (1984) The Pall ultipor breathing circuit filter: an efficient heat and moisture exchanger. International Anaesthesia Research Society, New York.

Cousins, D. (1988) Cost savings in IV therapy. *Care of the Critically Ill*, **4**, 1, 30-35.

DoH (1989) Working for Patients. Department of Health, London.

Gallagher, J. et al (1987) Contamination control in long-term ventilation. *Anaesthesia*, **42**, 476–81.

Griffiths, R. (Chair) (1983) NHS Management Enquiry. DHSS, London.

Johnson, A. (1985) Blueprint for the prevention and management of pressure sores. *Care; The British Journal of Rehabilitation and Tissue Viability*, **1**, 2, 8–13.

33

Resources review: product appraisal

Brenda Pottle , SRN, SCN, DN (Lond)
Senior Nurse, Specialist Research, East Surrey Health Authority

The nurses' involvement with purchasing decisions

In many purchasing decisions, the nurse on the ward or in the community has an important role. She uses many items of equipment and supplies every day, and also has the most detailed knowledge of the needs of the individual patient.

There has been, and often still is, a very large gap between the contracting supplies officer and the nurse on the ward, in the department, or in the community. This can widen if, for example, a company representative shows nurses products that are not available to them because there is a regional contracting system for purchase which excludes these products on grounds of cost or unsuitability. To be involved with decision-making at ward and regional levels nurses must be aware of the cost and be systematic in their appraisal of products. This information must then

PRODUCT APPRAISAL FORM

ITEM .... DURABLE ☐ DISPOSABLE ☐

MANUFACTURER/BRAND ....

Placement of contract for purchase of this item is being considered. If you have been using this product for not less than 3 months would you please assist the Supplies Department by completing this form.

When completed please return to ....

Name and Address of Unit
....
....
....

Type of Nursing e.g. "General"
....

Please tick the appropriate reply to these statements and questions	STRONGLY AGREE	AGREE	DISAGREE	STRONGLY DISAGREE	COMMENTS
1. This product is easy to use					
2. The quality is about right					
3. There are no major disadvantages					
4. It is suitable for the job					

5. Would you like this product to be available for ordering? YES ☐ NO ☐

6. If you know of an alternative product which is equally acceptable or better please give details

NAME ....

DESIGNATION ....

DATE ....

Figure 1. Product appraisal form.

be circulated to the appropriate people, and used effectively in reaching purchase decisions.

A system for product appraisal

A product appraisal system was devised by Doreen Norton by which to obtain basic facts about products in use (Norton, 1982). In such a survey, the nurses using the item are asked to complete a product appraisal form

PRODUCT APPRAISAL RESULTS			Ref. No. . . . .

ITEM . . . .   Date . . . .

MANUFACTURER/BRAND . . . .

Number P.A. Forms completed . . . .

Question 1-4:   4 × . . . . = ... (100%)

ANALYSIS OF RESULTS	A	B	Y	Z
	Strongly Agree	Agree	Disagree	Strongly Disagree
1. Product easy to use				
2. Quality about right				
3. No major disadvantages				
4. Suitable for the job				
TOTALS				

Total of **A + B** (favourable) . . . . (. . . . . . %)
Total of **Y + Z** (unfavourable) . . . . (. . . . . . %)

COMMON COMPLAINTS: in order of frequency of mention, with approximate number making comment.

	Number
. . . .	

5. Would like product available for ordering
      number . . . . percentage . . . .

ACTION TAKEN

Figure 2. Product appraisal result form.

(Figure 1), having had experience of using a product for three months. The opinion of nurses in different specialties can be included in the survey. The forms are then collated onto the product appraisal result form (Figure 2) for analysis and for use in decision making by the appropriate person or department.

This information gathered from the completed forms does not in itself constitute a rigorously researched evaluation of the product, but it does give a practical survey of the opinions of nurses and should reveal which products are suitable for purchase. The survey may indicate that further evaluation should be carried out.

This simple system can be used successfully in conjunction with a monitoring and costing exercise, for example examining three different types of wipe or cleaning tissue for incontinent patients.

Different manufacturers' products 1, 2, and 3 were each used for one week on one ward, over a period of three consecutive weeks. The product appraisal forms were completed by all nurses working on the ward during the trial and the results were collated onto the product appraisal result form. The results were as follows:

Product 1: A + B = 75% Y + Z = 25%
Product 2: A + B = 25% Y + Z = 75%
Product 3: A + B = 100%

This information was then forwarded to the contracting officer with the recommendation that **Product 3** should be selected for the regional contract (Smith; Unpublished Report).

A system for evaluation
More detailed evaluation of products may be required, and this will take more planning and research than the simple example just given.

To evaluate means "To determine significance or worth of usage by careful appraisal and study" (Webster, 1977). This means that there must be a commitment by staff, and in many circumstances patients, if the evaluation is to take place and be of value. A protocol must be written first to establish the criteria and the plan for the research. The process of product evaluation will be discussed in the following chapter.

Conclusion
Nurses have a vital role to play in appraising and evaluating resources, but the necessary research must be done in a systematic way and be carefully planned and properly documented. If the need for this discipline is recognized prior to an evaluation, this will surely stop the use of so-called "trials", in which one or two products are used with only one patient and then one product either praised or rejected. Incorrect decisions are often made as a result of inadequate or insufficiently documented factual information.

Nurses are increasingly involved with the decisions made on purchase. Ward budgeting is used in some hospitals and is a system that is likely to become more widely adopted in the future. One of the results of this system is that the ward sister or charge nurse may now be accountable for sizeable budgets for ward-based purchases. We owe it to our patients, our employers, our colleagues, and ourselves to make the best decisions.

References
Norton, D. (1982) What's in Store. Nursing Times, 1221.
Websters Dictionary (1977) Cassells, London.

34

Resources review: product evaluation

Brenda Pottle, SRN, SCM, DN (Lond)
Senior Nurse, Specialist Research, East Surrey Health Authority

Ward budgeting is a system that is used now in some hospitals and it is likely to be more widely adopted in the future. As a result, ward sisters may be accountable for sizeable budgets and they need to know how to make the best decisions on ward-based purchases of equipment and supplies.

A system for evaluation

In the previous chapter, the nurse's involvement with purchasing decisions was discussed and it was stressed that to be involved with decision making at ward and regional levels nurses must be aware of the costs and be systematic in their appraisal of products.

A simple system for product appraisal was illustrated which can provide a practical survey of nurses' opinions and reveal which products are suitable for purchase, but sometimes a more rigorous and detailed evaluation of products may be required, and this will take more planning and research.

To evaluate means ''To determine significance or worth of usage by careful appraisal and study'' (Webster, 1977). This means that there must be a commitment by staff, and in many circumstances patients, if the evaluation is to take place and be of value. A protocol must be written first to establish the criteria and the plan for the research.

Protocol for product evaluation

Purpose   There may be a number of reasons for undertaking product evaluation. A new product may have become available and an existing product in use over a number of years may not now be the best choice. Suitability of a product for a particular group of patients may be questioned. A comparison of products may be required and the cost-effectiveness of each may need to be evaluated.

Products to be used   All products to be included in the evaluation must be listed; details are taken from the manufacturer's specifications and literature.

Costs   These should be carefully defined and VAT included where applicable. The unit cost if a bulk purchase on a regional contract is made should also be known. If the product is not available on prescription, evaluation of it with patients in the community should be questioned, and the value of assessing these products considered carefully.

Literature search   Has anyone been down this path before? If so, what did their research cover and what were the results? Should those findings be tested again, or new methods employed?

Criteria to be tested   The manufacturer's literature can be used to draw up some of the questions that may be asked in finding out if it is suitable for the patient and the nurse to use. For example, a bandage to be evaluated has in its manufacturer's literature (Johnson and Johnson, 1984):
''Easy to apply and remove
Stick only to themselves
Easy for home and ward use
Aid compliance
Do not stick to hair or skin

Less discomfort and skin trauma
Tears easily to length without scissors
Conforms even on awkward sites
Extremely comfortable
Highly absorbent and permeable
Kind to skin
Fewer complications and fewer changes
Can be worn in water
Radiolucent''
   These statements can be used to draw up a questionnaire to assess the practical use of this product. Other criteria may include suitability for different groups of patients (such as children or the elderly) or the effectiveness of use by untrained personnel, who could include relatives.

Method of evaluation   The method used in the research must be planned out in detail. This should include the following:
Length of time in days, weeks, or months
Staff to be consulted
Numbers of patients and locations in hospital and/or community
Ethical issues
Instructions for using the products (company representatives could be
   involved here)
Design of the forms and questionnaires: Should these be piloted?
Monitoring the use of detailed forms. Is someone able to give the time
   personally to monitor the evaluation? Time and staff must be available
   to collate the results.

The research   With this planned out in detail, the forms and questionnaires devised (and if necessary piloted), and all the staff fully briefed, the information gathering can begin.

Results   Once the forms and questionnaires are collected, it takes time to collate the results. If a computer is available time can be saved, but monitoring forms and questionnaires must be designed before the research with full knowledge of the computer's potential in order to make best use of this resource. The limitations of the research must also be clearly identified (for example it may only be appropriate for one group of patients, cr one setting for care). The problems encountered while undertaking the research should also be reported.

Report   This needs to have all the details of the evaluation, limitations, problems encountered, costs, results, conclusions, and recommendations in a clear, typed format. Before writing the report, consideration must be given to its future use. It may be circulated to other nurses, administrators, or supplies officers only, or it may be made more widely available to the manufacturers or even for publication.

Reports are best written as soon as possible after the research is completed so that the most up-to-date information is made available to colleagues. Imposing a deadline for the completion of the report may help with this. The report must be circulated to appropriate colleagues, including the nurses involved with the evaluation and the budget holder.

Conclusion

Incorrect decisions on purchasing are often made as a result of inadequate or insufficiently documented factual information. Nurses have a vital role to play in appraising and evaluating resources, and the necessary research must be done in a systematic way, with careful planning and proper documentation. Recognition of the need for such discipline prior to an evaluation should avoid the use of so-called "trials", when one or two products are used with only one patient and then one product is praised or rejected on this basis.

References

Johnson and Johnson Ltd (1984) New Secure and Secure Forte Literature.
Norton, D. (1982) What's in Store. *Nursing Times*, 1221.
Websters Dictionary (1977) Cassells, London.

35

Measuring product performance

Doreen Norton, OBE, MSc, SRM, FRCN
*Retired; formerly Nursing Research Liaison Officer, South West Thames RHA and
Professor of Gerontological Nursing, Case Western Reserve University, Cleveland, Ohio*

Evaluation means measuring performance against prescribed criteria. The first step to conducting a reliable trial of a product is writing the prescription for the performance, as these criteria are the basis for planning the data-collecting form or questionnaire to be used in the trial. 'Measuring' means the information sought and obtained must be capable of interpretation in numerical form.

This article offers guidance on these aspects of product performance trials. It is written in terms of a single product but the same principles apply when two or more of the same kind are subjected to comparative

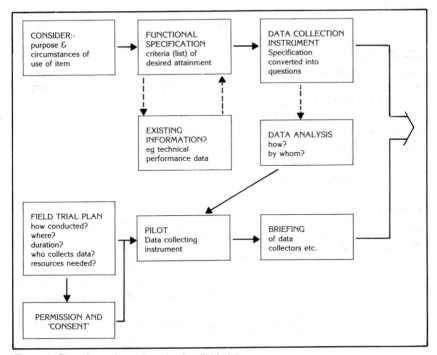

Figure 1. Steps in equipment evaluation field trial.

evaluation of performance. Any field trial must be systematically planned (Figure 1) and based on scientific principles.

Criteria prescription

What is the purpose of the product and the general circumstances of its use? Write a concise statement answering these two questions (Figure 2). This is not always easy, but worthwhile because it focuses the mind and throws up issues which can easily be missed through familiarity with the nursing tasks involved in using such an item.

a) Roughly list all the functions and properties which, ideally, are desired of the product in fulfilment of its purpose and in the circumstances of its use. Note any information supplied by the manufacturer, particularly technical specifications, and adjust the list accordingly.

Figure 2. Criteria specifications.

ITEM: Disposable theatre cap.
PURPOSE: To keep hair enclosed for (a) hygenic reasons and (b) uninhibited vision and movement.
MAIN SITUATIONS OF USE: Operating theatres and intensive care units.

REQUIREMENTS	EXPLANATION AND CONSTRAINTS
MATERIAL 1. Shall be reasonably non-generating of static electricity.	(i) Cap worn in the presence of anaesthetic gases.
2. Shall allow ventilation.	(ii) Operating theatres have a temperature of 18-24°C and humidity of 40-50%; therefore the head covering must not impede heat evaporation from the scalp nor generate its own heat.
3. Shall remain intact when handled (donning of cap) and throughout use.	(iii) Must not disintegrate, stretch or contract under conditions of heat and humidity (ii).
4. Shall be non-irritating to skin.	(iv) Length of time in contact with skin (v) and environmental conditions (ii) increase risk of skin irritation.
THE CAP 5. Should be reasonably light in weight and softly flexible.	(v) Cap may be worn up to eight hours and therefore should not give awareness of weight or rigidity in the interests of comfort.
6. Shall be easy to put on.	(vi) —
. . .etc. . .	. . .etc. . .

This example of prescribed criteria was developed as an exercise with a group of nurses from East Surrey Health Authority in 1982.

b) Now examine each entry critically, with a view to revising the list by deletions and modifications. Extract and record separately, for example, any factor which would require to be tested other than in the field trial, such as a bacterial test in a laboratory. Bear in mind throughout that demands made of the product must be realistic and that each stated requirement will later involve framing questions to ascertain if, and to what extent it is met in performance of the product.

c) Assemble the remaining entries into some form of order, eg grouping of related factors or an appropriate logical sequence.

d) Against each entry, record into which of three categories it falls — essential (it shall), desirable (should), permissible (may). The terms in brackets will apply when finalising the wording of the criteria.

e) Prepare for the revised list by dividing a large sheet of paper into two sections, one headed **Requirements** and the other **Explanation and Constraints.** Now comes the brain-teasing part — not to be rushed! It is advisable to study the example (Figure 2) at this stage.

f) Make each entry under 'Requirements' a precise statement in terms of functional performance. (Do not specify design or materials — express only the properties required of them.) Try to make the statements in the positive, ie what the product must, should or may do, rather than what it must not do. (The 'must nots' should become apparent under the other section heading). Under 'Explanation and constraints' record information which clarifies the entry opposite. Indeed, it is advisable to work through such information and assemble any extrinsic facts necessary before attempting to finalise the wording of the statement of Requirements.

Data collecting instrument

Whatever the plan decided for conduct of the trial, the criteria have to be converted into some form of questioning of observers about the product's performance under working conditions.

The kind of questioning varies with the nature of the requirement; it can be a direct question or a statement for agreement/disagreement. In either, a 'yes/no' type of answering may be appropriate for some factors but for others allowance usually has to be made in the data collecting instrument for recording degrees of the product's compliance with the requirement. An even number of degrees (say, four or six) is preferable to an uneven number (say, three or five) as this allows for a balance of degrees towards satisfactory and unsatisfactory and avoids the less helpful 'middle of the road' reply. The more degrees there are the more refined the information obtained but it is often necessary to strike a compromise between the amount and sophistication of information sought and the resources available for collecting and analysing the data.

Scoring of points

To achieve measurement of a product's performance, a weighted value of points is allocated to the optional replies to a question. Maximum points are given for total compliance with the requirement (completely satisfactory) to nil for no compliance (completely unsatisfactory). The number of intervals between depends on the number of degrees of compliance allowed for, eg four degrees will be in the order of 3,2,1,0 in value, but in any event the points' 'weighting' must be proportionately equal in their graduation steps.

Measurable analysis

The sum of the maximum points obtainable to all questions gives the 'ideal' performance score. The points scored by the product are then totalled and this figure calculated as a percentage of the 'ideal' score.

Example: Ideal score 58; obtained score 38.

$$\frac{3800}{58} = 65.5 \text{ per cent compliance with the criteria.}$$

If the product is a disposable or requires treatment before being used again (such as laundering) it may be decided to record observations at each incident of use rather than to collect data at the end of the trial period. In this case, the formula for analysis is to multiply the 'ideal' score by the number of times the item was used and the total of the obtained scores calculated as a percentage.

Example: Ideal score 58 x 110 incidents of use = 6380 max.
Obtained score total = 4125.

$$\frac{412500}{6380} = 64.6 \text{ per cent compliance with the criteria.}$$

Refinement of results   Irrespective of when data are collected, a refinement of results can be obtained if desirable. Namely, by isolating those requirements earlier identified as essential (shall) and applying the same procedure to their respective total of maximum points possible and the obtained score. It may be decided that the product is unacceptable if it fails to satisfy any one of these requirements or achieves less than, say, 90 per cent, in respect of these, however well it rated overall.

Comparative evaluations   When two or more products of the same kind (and used in the same way) are to receive a field trial to determine the most suitable, the principle is the same as for a single product. That is, the performance of each is measured against the prescribed criteria (and not simply compared with each other) and rated accordingly. All, however, must be subjected to the same trial conditions and, preferably, using the same observers.

It was mentioned at the outset that reliable information is the key to products being designed suitable for purpose and acceptable in the work situation. Manufacturers are starved of such information, and weaknesses in the design of products can be generally attributed to the failure of health care professionals to produce user-specifications. A performance criteria drawn-up for trial purposes and a user-specification are one and the same, so performance criteria made known to manufacturers can influence future design for the better. In any event, a full report of a product trial (including details of the methods) should always be sent to the manufacturer concerned.

References

Buckles, A.M. (1980) How should we dispose of our used needles and syringes? *Nursing Times*, **76**, 34, Journal of Infection Control Nursing, ICNA, 5–11.
An evaluation of four different types of containers for the disposal of sharps which serves as a good example of a comparative type of field trial using product performance measurement.

Norton, D. (1978) Equipment fit for purpose. *Nursing Times*, **74**, 19, Occasional Papers, 73–76.
Describes in detail the principles of specifying and evaluating equipment and for conducting field trials.

INDEX